VOICES OF DONOR CONCEPTION

(VOLUME I)

BEHIND CLOSED DOORS:

MOVING BEYOND SECRECY AND SHAME

EDITED BY MIKKI MORRISSETTE

IN AFFILIATION WITH THE DONOR SIBLING REGISTRY

For updates and further insights stemming from this book series, see

www.VoicesOf Donor Conception.com

Book and cover design: Mary Leir

First printing, December 2006

ISBN: 978-0-9772042-1-2

"The measure of a man's intelligence is the number of conflicting ideas

he can hold in his mind at the same time."

— F. Scott Fitzgerald

CONTENTS

INTRODUCTION
BY MIKKI MORRISSETTE

The genesis for this book started out innocently enough at a symposium in Toronto, where I gave a speech about the fact that donor insemination is the method to motherhood for roughly half of the hundreds of Choice Moms/single mothers by choice that I know.

During the two-day event, organized by Diane Allen of Infertility Network, I met Wendy and Ryan Kramer, Olivia Montuschi, Eric Schwartzman and Rebecca Hamilton—all people you will meet in this book. Each of them offered unique and important perspectives on a multimillion-dollar industry that affects tens of thousands of new lives every year, yet tends to operate without much public discussion. The stories that do trickle out through the media tend to have a narrow focus: half-siblings who have met, neurological diseases shared by offspring of the same anonymous donor, single women who choose their child's "father" from an online donor catalog.

For the typical donor-conceived family, however, there are many complex and deeply personal stories not shared in public. The infertile husband who is (secretly) afraid of being less of a parent to his child, or of being perceived as less of a man in the family. The parents who fear that if their child grows up knowing about the existence of a donor it will usurp their place of authority. The child who notices that "you take after…" comparisons get awkwardly clipped short of discussion involving one side the family, and is afraid to ask why.

Indeed, many families feel so protective of their privacy regarding donor conception that fear seems to take over. Fear of what people would think if they knew. Fear of what impact it will have on the child to know—or to not know.

Donors, too, tend to operate in secret. Many do not tell loved ones in later years that they offered up part of themselves on a regular basis so that children could be created to people they don't know.

As a result of all the fear and secrecy surrounding donor conception, tens of thousands of kids grow up thinking — whether the words are spoken or not — that there was something "wrong," or "odd," or simply shameful about their birth.

But really, given that thousands of families have turned to reproductive technology over the years, why should donor conception still be considered shameful? Why should a single mother, or a couple struggling with infertility, pass along anything to their child other than the message that "a deep and abiding desire to love and nurture a child led me/us to take great lengths to bring you into the world."

Such openness doesn't magically whisk away issues of donor conception that some children will feel (Who is the donor? How am I like him/her?). But it relieves parents of a terrible burden. And in so doing, frees up the hundreds of thousands of people affected by donor conception in the United States alone to really talk about how to become better served as a community.

> *There are many issues about donor conception that can—*
> *sometimes easily—be tackled, simply by getting out from*
> *behind closed doors and talking about them as a group.*

For example, should donor-conceived kids be entitled to have updated medical histories of their donors, for future use in screening cancers and other diseases that are known to have a genetic base?

Should the number of offspring to one donor be limited more carefully than it is today? Or should more strenuous screening of an elite pool of donors be encouraged so that parents have a better sense of the genetic health of the "product" they are buying?

About This Book

The people who have been asked to contribute to this book all have a healthy, unashamed approach to donor conception. They tend to have strong opinions about what could be done better—and they don't always agree with each other. They were selected because their ability to be open, articulate and balanced serves to move the industry a step further in engaging discussion about how improvements can be made so that the needs of parents, donors AND offspring can be met.

In this book we hear from an infertile husband who is honest about his insecurities as the non-biological parent. We hear from a donor who is in the early stages of welcoming contact with one of his offspring into the life he has already created for himself, which includes five children of his own. We hear from experts about how, when, and why to tell children the story of their conception. We hear advice and insight from three donor-conceived offspring—one a mother of two—for the next generation of parents. And we get seven specific recommendations for reform in the industry, offered by a parent, an adult offspring, and a donor.

This book is largely being marketed by Wendy Kramer, co-founder with her son of The Donor Sibling Registry. She has been proactively working on advocating in the industry since her son Ryan was 10 and asking questions that, until then, she had not realized would be important. She has made it her mission to make anyone who will listen aware of the fact that kids will want to know more about their donor as extensions of themselves. And rather than wish she had never told Ryan, when he was two, about his origins in a doctor's office, she is a strong advocate for encouraging natural curiosity as a way to bond and create deeper respect between parent and child.

Wendy did not choose what topics or which writers would be included in this volume, although two of the contributors came from contacts she has made over the years. She did help fund the production of this book, as part of her ongoing effort to help more families take pride in their donor conception roots.

Voices of Donor Conception book series

As part of the ongoing discussion, I hope to publish several other titles in a series called Voices of Donor Conception. Forthcoming topics might cover: Do's and don'ts of making contact with donors and half-siblings; the anonymity and open-identity options; what we should know about genetics; issues specific to egg donation (which is not covered adequately in this volume).

As editor of the series, it is not my intent to oversimplify the issues. Not everyone agrees on how to handle anonymity, disclosure, and record-keeping. I want to reflect that in future volumes. I encourage readers to contact me directly with their stories at **DCVoices@gmail. com**. As with the hundreds of Choice Moms I have been in contact with over the years, all stories will be handled confidentially.

In the meantime, the hope with *Behind Closed Doors: Moving Beyond Secrecy and Shame* is to help move readers through an open door to the other side, where everything is not simple, but it is honest. Where infertility is not a matter of shame, but a physiological issue—like the diabetic whose body doesn't produce insulin—that affects 1 out of 10 couples. Where adoption and donor conception are merely methods to parenthood. Where entitlement to parent is not limited to whether one's eggs or sperm were used to create a new life. Where children grow up knowing as much as they choose to about their genetic inheritance, as a healthy extension of understanding who they are.

In Gay Becker's book *Elusive Embryo: How Women and Men Approach New Reproductive Technologies* (University of California Press, 2000), she writes that the biological focus in the United States is misplaced. Creating a life is not simply a matter of biology, but of raising a child who is connected emotionally with family, encouraged to develop a strong identity, and integrated into the larger community.

The goal of this book is to help move past the biology, and move us toward working collaboratively so that our children are empowered and encouraged to develop their strongest potential as individuals who are integrated into a full community of loved ones and kin.

In the Footsteps of Our Cousins

"I think the best thing we all can do is [educate ourselves].
Read good articles, online publications and books. Attend
informational sessions and really listen and don't let your
normal, understandable desire to have a child obscure your
ability to assimilate what you're learning. When you're
better educated about anything, it does usually lead to better
outcomes. The effect is that you have better-informed parents
who understand their sons' and daughters' needs, who are
more respectful of their backgrounds, and who are more
thoughtful about the specific issues in their lives. That sounds
like a good start to me."

— Adam Pertman, executive director of the Evan B. Donaldson
Adoption Institute, in an interview about adoption with American
Fertility Association's Carolyn Berger

VOICES OF PARENTS

Some of us need help to conceive — due to physiology, or due to the lack of a partner.

With this kind of help, points out Diane Ehrensaft, author of *Mommies, Daddies, Donors, Surrogates: Answering Tough Questions and Building Families* (The Guilford Press, 2005), comes inevitable struggles with issues such as:

Power — What do I want people to know about my child's origins? What do I want my child to know?

Ownership — Whose child is this anyway? If I didn't help make it, is it mine? If I did help make it, is it more mine?

Collaboration — How does the birth other fit into my family?

In this section, we hear the realities of donor conception, from the view of an infertile husband, a long-time donor who is making contact with one of his offspring, and two experts who have talked with hundreds of donor-conceived families.

CHAPTER 1

"HI, MY NAME IS ERIC, AND I'M INFERTILE"

BY ERIC SCHWARTZMAN

There aren't a lot of support groups for men like me. Mainly because not many of us are willing to publicly admit to being infertile, since it implies a lesser strain of masculinity.

In actuality, infertility is something that is quite out of our control. In some cases we were severely injured (like the guy who was kicked by a bull at age 13). Others had a childhood illness that rendered them impotent. In my case—you probably don't want to know the details—I was born with testes that were not fully descended. I had an operation at the age of eight, and was given a variety of hormone treatments to get them in place.

When I was an adult, I was advised to get a basic semen analysis. The diagnosis: non-obstructive azoospermia. A fancy way of saying that I had no functional sperm to swim anywhere.

I learned this six months before I was to be married. The doctor bluntly stated, "You'll never have natural children and should just accept it." My fiancée nearly jumped across his desk to kill him for the insensitive nature of his diagnosis and advice.

For me, marriage and child-raising go hand-in-hand. I'm an avid genealogist, so family history and genes mean a lot to me. I was absolutely crushed by the news that I could never have kids "the normal way." I even gave my fiancée an out, if she wanted to call off the wedding and find a new man who could impregnate her. (She almost throttled me for that suggestion, too.)

We got married, and put the issues aside for a few years. Financially and emotionally, we needed to build up our reserves before deciding on our options.

Eventually we decided to go for the Big Solution. A cycle of IVF and ICSI at Cornell. They were going to do a testicular biopsy on me to see if there was sperm hiding in the corners that they could implant in my wife's egg. We were advised to pick an anonymous donor as a backup source in case they had no sperm to use from my body.

We were so hopeful about the procedure that the potential use of a donor wasn't something we ever focused on. We simply looked at the two biggest sperm banks that were recommended by the clinic. No one talked to us about how to select a donor, or what the use of a donor might mean to our family.

Primarily we wanted to find a donor that shared my religious background—Jewish—which severely limited our choices.

We briefly discussed using a known donor from my family or friends, but instinctively felt uncomfortable with the idea. I have no male siblings or male cousins I felt comfortable asking. My wife nixed any thoughts of asking my father as too weird—the issue of my being a half sibling to my own son was also too strange.

Under time pressure to pick someone before the cycle, we selected a donor in a rushed fashion. We were working under the expectation that his sperm would never be needed. We bought only two vials.

And in fact, the biopsy did find a few of my sperm tucked away, resulting in three embryos. Unfortunately, none of the embryos "took." So our first attempt failed. Six months later, giving my body time to recover from the first biopsy, we tried the same procedure. Also without success.

My wife vetoed the idea of a third attempt. It was a taxing procedure for me physically. We agreed that donor insemination should become Plan A. Since there were no remaining vials of our Jewish donor, we took a new look at finding the "perfect" donor. This time some of the reality set in of what we were attempting.

The search takes on a strange meaning when you know you are picking someone to impregnate your wife.

Several IUI attempts with donor #2 failed. Now the panic was that we would never become parents through conception. One of the reasons we weren't enamored with adoption as an option was that we wanted more control over neo-natal care. We wanted to know that my wife was doing everything she could to create a healthy environment for the fetus during each stage of pregnancy. We wouldn't feel that level of control with adoption.

Yet as we became more focused on the use of donor sperm, we realized there were many fears we'd never considered before. We had his bios and medical history, but who could assure us that the donor was telling the complete truth? Who could assure us that he knew his family's medical history, as a young student? Who could assure us that the screening tests conducted by the bank were complete enough?

We were planning to introduce a foreign substance into my wife's body and we realized we only had a limited amount of information about the donor and possible genetic frailties that would be passed onto our children.

But blindly, while fighting our pain of infertility, we pushed forward and accepted the risks.

Eventually we switched to another fertility clinic. Whether it was new luck or a change of venues, we finally succeeded in our quest to become parents. Our son was conceived, not in a romantic setting on a starry night, but during IUI cycle #7. A few years later, using the same donor, our daughter was born.

When the Fears Began

It was during my wife's first pregnancy that I began to worry about what using DI really meant. That a third party, who I didn't know, was now indirectly responsible for my child's creation. That biologically that man was my son's father. And that, simply put, I was jealous of what the donor's sperm was able to accomplish that my own body could not.

I will admit to some wild fears, including:
- my son would instinctively know that I was an imposter;
- he would not want me to hold him from birth;
- our families would always whisper in hushed voices that he was not really mine and would smile politely at family gatherings;
- if my kids were to someday meet the donor, they might decide he was the only daddy they wanted.

None of our friends or family knew the difficulties we were having trying to conceive. It was only after telling our parents of the pregnancy that we told them about using donor insemination.

We still hadn't thought through when or how we would tell our children—there was only so much we could think about at once—but we did both agree that, however we did it, they would be told at an early age. We'd read a few books to help us make that decision.

I know some men struggle with the irrational fear that donor insemination is the equivalent of their wife being unfaithful to them. Or that their wife, if given the chance, would run off with the "father" of their children—or at the very least fantasize about him. Or the concern that he won't be able to love a child that does not feel like his. Or the worry that the wife will see the child as more hers than his. Or the fear that the wife will simply see him as less of a man because he couldn't impregnate her.

But to be honest, my thoughts were too focused on the possibility that my children would reject me.

I had read in the few books available that someday a teenager would rebel and yell, "You aren't my real father." That I knew I would get over, hurtful as it might be at the time. In fact, I expect it. But what I am really afraid of is that my teenager will run away from home to find the "real" dad.

Sure, over time, they will love me as their dad, but knowing that the decision to use DI could inflict such feelings of loss scares the hell out of me more than anything else.

I don't regret choosing DI, but it was my choice, not theirs, and this fear is my greatest.

My Education

To help me work through some of my fears, I started writing an online blog, "Life as Dad to Donor Insemination Kids." I also helped launch a Yahoo discussion support group called "DI Dads," which I now moderate.

As a result, I was asked to participate at a symposium sponsored by the Toronto-based Infertility Network. As one of the few "DI dads" who was public, I was asked to speak from my perspective on the use of donor insemination. Little did I know that attending that seminar, in October 2005, would lead to my greatest fear: That I had unintentionally hurt my children.

At that conference I met several adults who were conceived from donor insemination. I began to see how DI is a one-sided answer to the pain of infertile adults like myself, but does not take into account the eventual emotional needs of the donor-conceived child.

I learned by listening that by using DI, my wife and I had in effect intentionally cut off our children from their genetic and ethnic past. We had cut them off from one-half of their identity.

The individuals I met varied in age, and were affected in different degrees by the choices their parents had made to conceive them. The emotional pain evoked by some of these individuals was almost overwhelming for me to experience.

Thus far I had been consumed with fears about my wife and I in dealing with infertility, disappointments at failed attempts, physical and financial and mental issues, and having a stranger produce my child. But now a new concern had sprung up that I'd never considered before. My own children could someday feel the kind of pain that the adults I was meeting felt.

I was asked if, in hindsight, after learning their stories, would I still use DI? My answer was the truth, although I'm sure it was seen as a cop-out. I could not answer. I knew we were not planning on having more kids. I had a much larger bounty of information about the donor we used than did the families of most of these individuals. We had medical health bios of him and his family, a toddler picture, a voice recording of him on CD, etc.

The people I heard from at the seminar had nothing. And the pain of that showed.

My response was that perhaps my kids' experience would be different. Perhaps they would not share this loss as deeply.

But I haven't shaken the things I learned that weekend. My biggest fear continues to be that despite all the information we do have, the desire we put into conceiving, the thought we've given to telling them at a young age—will it be enough? Despite all this, will they feel that terrible sense of loss and incompletion? Will they need answers we cannot give them? Will they reject me, not because I am their non-biological father, but because I did not enable them to know who they are by looking into the face of their biological father?

My goals since that seminar have been to learn as much as I can to be able to discuss these issues with my kids when the time comes.

A Day-to-Day DI Life

As a blogger dealing with DI every day through my writing, the issue is always in my mind. Little by little, via my postings, I feel I give away more of my anonymity about who I am, while I learn nothing more of the donor.

My day-to-day fears are that the donor will come looking for my kids to reclaim as his own. That his "DNA" identification card will give him full rights to the kids.

Of course, I know that legally their mother and I are their only parents under New York State law, but the thought of being supplanted by an interested donor scares me. As it does many "social fathers" like me, I now know.

Medically, my family didn't improve the gene pool. The medical histories we have show the donor's family to be as messed up as mine historically, with many of the classic malaises experienced by my clan. The kids will forever have to memorize these histories and, when asked for their "father's" info, answer with this knowledge, forever reinforcing their unnatural status as my children. Granted, having this info is better than not having it, but it creates a periodic reminder that I fear could bring them pain.

My son has known since he was two years old that a donor helped mommy and daddy create him (and later his sister). For most of his young life we have minimized the donor's role to just that act. But in truth he plays a much bigger role, whose impact we can't yet see, because his unknown DNA is one half of my children.

My concern now is imposing my views and fears and wants on these kids, and not allowing them to make their own decisions as to who the donor is to them. What I need to do is to teach them all I know, but to trust their intuition about what is right for them, and to help them get to a point of comfort so that they can live their lives without feeling a giant gap.

In short, my greatest fear now is what emotional harm I may have set them up for.

CHAPTER 2

MY LIFE AS A DONOR,
NO LONGER ANONYMOUS
BY KIRK MAXEY

In 1979, my first wife suggested that I become a sperm donor. She was a nurse, and introduced me to an ob/gyn in Michigan who did infertility treatment. When he needed a specimen, he told my wife, who told me. I donated perhaps a few dozen times.

This was the old-fashioned version of semen donation. One that no longer exists. I suspect that it led to perhaps 10,000 births per year. There were no tests of any kind. You became a donor because you were personally known to the physician who was performing the procedure, and he could vouch for your general health and disease-free state. I think most of the donors were married men.

Three months after I moved to start medical school, I was recruited to become a donor by partners in another reproduction clinic. I assumed they were referred to me by the previous doctor. This time there were some tests. I had a karyotype (the standard arrangement of pairs of chromosomes that can be used to determine aberrations, as well as sex of the individual). And I was asked for a brief family health history. I was not asked anything about my hobbies or interests or accomplishments. It was clear that they intended to tell the mothers virtually nothing about me. I merely supplied information about my height, weight, hair, eyes and blood type.

Bit by bit, medical tests were required to stay in the program, for

HIV, then Hep B, CMV, chlamydia, gonorrhea, syphilis. In the end it was like getting certified for entry into heaven. Hard physical proof that I never did anything nasty or caught any bad bugs.

A nurse called frequently in the evenings to set up donations. This was another feature of the old methods of donor insemination: fresh semen was used within hours of donation. The events were carefully timed and orchestrated. I would get specific windows of time during which I had to donate. It was important to be very punctual, or else one risked running into the semen recipient while visiting the clinic.

You can imagine the difficulty of having to produce a specimen on cue at 3:35 p.m., which might be just after having been in a class about gross anatomy.

Today, of course, a donor is free to produce semen specimens whenever he feels like it, because there is no urgency. They will all be frozen and quarantined for six months to undergo testing. This puts the donor in control of how many times a week he will donate, and how much money he will try to earn. In my case, I was always called on the phone by the clinic. I never "decided" that it was time to get another $20 for a semen sample. (And in those days we weren't paid much more than that.)

The impact on me of these repeated requests was substantial and positive. For one, it was flattering. Since I was 'asked back" for 15 years, I imagined that some combination of the patient's preferences and the clinic's judgment indicated that I was a "good" donor. I expected that the doctors were monitoring the outcomes of these pregnancies and saw high conception rates with patients, or vigorous and healthy babies. It never once occurred to me that I was simply a reliable donor who was earning them a lot of money.

In more recent years, however, I realized that this "good" thing that I imagined about my donor activity was a mirage. I was appalled when I learned that there was no monitoring in place. The doctor I worked with did not know how many kids had been born using my donations, or where they lived. For the first time, I had a very bad, sinking feeling that I had been used. Perhaps for hundreds of offspring.

I am the father of five kids, including one stepdaughter, and I continue to have a quiet but steady longing to know something about these other offspring. Just to know how many there are, how they are doing, what they enjoy. And especially whether they are healthy and safe. I also strongly believe I should be available to answer any questions they might have about me.

Recently, my quiet longing to know something about my offspring led to contact with a teenager who came from one of my donations.

Meeting my offspring

I'll call her Willow.

For her, I think it was a sudden, confusing turn of events to learn that she was donor conceived and—a few days later—to make contact with me. Her mother had suddenly told her about her conception, shortly before she graduated from high school. Three days later she found me listed on the DSR website and sent me an e-mail saying "I think you're my biological father."

It was all too easy, and at first she didn't trust it. She wanted to have some confirming tests run. But I think as we started to chat over e-mail, she began to feel sort of a kinship, and her talk of wanting to be tested drifted away.

For me, I had been thinking about these possible offspring for 25 years. I always half expected that eventually, I would meet one. When more than a year went by after I listed on the DSR and no one matched, it was actually very disappointing. I had "match envy." So when I got her e-mail, tears really did come to my eyes. I was happy just for myself—that I found one of my "lost kids."

What made it better was her profound sense of relief to have found her bio-dad. I think what her Mom told her really threw her for a loop, so it was important for her to have "that nice man who donated" available immediately as a real person, rather than a huge question mark. In the end, she told me I was the best graduation present that she got.

As with most donor-conceived children, I don't think that she believes this was a great way to do things. It is another one of those fundamental failures of the adults who run the world.

She happens to live just 20 minutes from me, and the same distance from my oldest son, who is just five years older. Interestingly, my son isn't curious enough to meet her. His version is, "Well Dad, I support you and everything, but I'm really busy with school right now."

At home with my younger kids and my wife, there is a polite distance that we practice. I don't talk with Willow on the phone when I'm home. I don't announce it when she wants to meet me somewhere. My family has taken a fairly cool attitude towards her—from their perspective, she's connected to me, but not to them.

Although it's complex, I admittedly do feel paternal toward her. I feel protective of her. I don't want her feelings to be hurt. And there are times when I feel like I need to give her words of advice.

Of course, as any parent would be, you are off in the background anyway after they turn 18. They only chat with you when they want to. They have their own agenda and their own goals. So I feel very much like any parent in that sort of second-class position does.

The fact that donor - offspring relationships are certainly possible, and come with some emotional burdens, cannot be taken lightly. For that reason, I would disqualify as a donor anyone who expresses negativity towards parent-child relationship in general. Anyone should be disqualified from the very start as a donor if he says something to the effect, "I don't really like kids, and don't ever want the burden of raising them or having to deal with their issues..."

Yes, most donors are young, and aren't ready for parenting yet, but they need to know from the start that there will be offspring. Young women and men who will someday want to know at least something about their donor father. They will want to be acknowledged. Some will want to ask questions about personality, fears, emotions. The donor had better be prepared both from an emotional and a maturity standpoint to accept that position when the time comes—even "anonymous" donors like I was. Times are changing, and kids who want to know will be smart enough technology-wise to find out, with the help of DNA analysis that gets more sophisticated every year.

Negotiating contact between Willow and I hasn't been simple. But we seem to like each other. We both like to write, and have exchanged pieces of creative writing with each other. We both speak some French. We both seem to approve, in general, of the other, which makes our relations with each other easier.

But the one glaring contradiction that I can see with allowing donors unlimited offspring (see my reform suggestion at the end of the book) is that, in the end, you can be stretched beyond your limits. It just does not seem natural to my existing family that a new person who wants to take up my time should pop out of the woodwork. And they might get downright angry if ten or more of them did.

As it is, I play a very delicate role of mediator, trying to see Willow when she would like to meet, but also making sure that this is okay with her Mom and Dad, and also not a disruption to my own kids. My younger son, for example, would not take it kindly if I missed his soccer game to go meet Willow at the mall.

It is difficult specifically because I did not know Willow, or that she had any interest in me, until last year. By then I was 50, and she had already lived 18 years without knowing I existed. If this had been allowed to develop more gradually (for both me, and my own family) I think it would have been much less disruptive.

So, I am making a plug here for early notification of donors that they have a child. And the offspring should know, by the time they are 5 or 6, some basic information about their donor so the relationships can develop slowly, over time, as they are supposed to.

Chapter 3

How to Tell

by Olivia Montuschi

Telling children about donor conception makes adults feel uncomfortable. Even those parents who strongly believe that their children have a right to the information get butterflies in their stomach at the thought of actually talking with their children about how their family came into being.

It is not difficult to understand why this is so. Donor conception is not the first choice of any heterosexual couple and few single women when it comes to family making. This method of conception almost always follows loss, grief and probably a long period of heartache.

My husband and I were lucky that we did not have to struggle over whether to tell our two children. We both felt from the start that deception about their genetic origins was not a good basis for family relationships. But we did wonder how and what we would tell them as there was no help available 20 years ago.

I thought I was comfortable talking with others about our children's beginnings—until a surprising amount of anxiety was revealed when I stumbled and stuttered over the words when it was time to tell our son's schoolteachers. (I needn't have worried. No one has ever shown us or our children anything other than warmth and support.)

We started to 'tell' our eldest child when he began asking questions about how babies are made at the age of four. I don't remember beginning to tell our daughter, as the subject was around our family by then and information trickled down. But we did have to be careful to check what she understood. It was clear at one point that she thought I knew her donor, as I had referred to him as a 'nice man.'

Over more than a decade I have talked with thousands of families that are affected by donor conception. All of my work with the Donor Conception Network has evolved from those early experiences with my own children.

Where the Shame Comes From

Infertility may be perceived as something to be ashamed of, which brings stigma to the man, woman or couple involved. Parents may feel less masculine or womanly because of their infertility and not wish to reveal their condition to the world by 'telling' others.

And there are the sexual associations with making babies, and the guilt of unsuccessful lovemaking and infertility.

Male infertility has often been (wrongly) confused with lack of virility. Sperm donation involves sexual stimulation and has long had overtones of seediness. Many adults did not receive sex education. It is hardly surprising that trying to explain to their own children about unassisted conception, let alone donor conception, is so difficult.

"Why would I want to do this and how on earth would I go about it even if I did?"

If educating our children about how they were born is not difficult enough, there are many other reasons parents put it off—or decide not to attempt it at all.

Some parents explain that they do not want to 'tell' because they think the information will confuse their child, or they worry that their child will be rejected by others, or that their child will reject the non-genetic mom or dad. Others are adamant that genetics don't matter and that, 'we're going to love her to bits anyway so why does she need to know?'

Of course, if genetics really was unimportant to the family, then sharing the information about the non-genetic element of the story would not be a big deal at all.

All these conflicting and confusing feelings often lead parents to believe that 'telling' would only upset relationships in the family, and so keeping the secret is better for all concerned. These feelings, however, belong to the adults concerned. They are not shared by children who come into the world without assumptions about what being donor conceived means.

> *It is the emotional climate in which they are reared, and the experiences they have, both inside and outside the family, that will lead them to either feel proud and comfortable with who they are, or to share their parents' feelings of loss and shame.*

Emotions connected with shame and stigma, along with profound shock and betrayal of trust, have been talked about by some donor-conceived adults who were told or who found out about their donor conception later in life. The same adults also talk about living with a terrible sense of something being wrong in the family as they grew up. This often led to low self-esteem and difficulties in finding their place in the world.

The Difference That Confidence Can Make

My 14 years of experience as director of the Donor Conception Network has revealed to me that parental confidence in using donor conception as a method of family creation—as well as openness with children from an early age—are the best predictors of warm, trusting family relationships.

When the family has an open atmosphere, it allows parents to share their feelings with each other—not denying or pushing away the occasional sadness for children they could not create together—right alongside the enormous love they share for the children they do have.

This recognition of the possibility of mixed feelings creates the conditions for children to develop their own feelings about being donor conceived, and to receive understanding and support from their parents whenever they might need it. In this way, openness breeds honesty, depth of feeling and trust over the years.

Secrecy, on the other hand, shuts down the possibility of discussion about the inevitable emotions about donor conception. Leaving emotions and issues unspoken does not mean they don't exist.

Secrecy also prevents the acknowledgment of mixed feelings, and breeds only fear and bewilderment. It also takes up huge energy. Avoiding a family chat about who looks like who, or who shares similar habits, is simply felt by children at a subconscious level.

'Telling' is actually easier than not telling

Once parents have overcome, or at least acknowledged and begun to address their own fears, then starting the donor conception story very early in a child's life gives parents the chance to practice the language. It also gives children the opportunity to incorporate 'their story' into their development.

Simple language is the key to building, brick by brick, an understanding of how a child came to be part of the family. Many of the roughly 1,000 families in our Network begin to chat with their child about their origins when they are just days old. You can use whatever words you like with a baby so long as they convey love and pride.

When parents talk with their baby in this way, then it is very natural to continue to look for 'hooks' to hang further information on. For example, if an aunt is expecting a baby, parents can talk about how 'babies grow in mommy's tummies, but sometimes mommies and daddies need some help to make a baby.'

If a journey is taking a family past the clinic where conception took place, parents can comment as matter-of-factly as if they were passing a fire station: 'That's where Mommy went when we needed some help to have you.'

Children's stories or programs on TV about families can all become opportunities to talk about the different ways that families come into being. There are now many specially written storybooks for young children to help them understand about donor conception. A popular idea is to include space for the child's photo at the end of the story. Many families create their own specialized scrapbook to tell the story.

Typical Ages and Stages

Around the age of four, children might start to ask where babies come from and how they themselves were made. This is part of a child's normal curiosity about the mechanics of human bodies. It has nothing to do with sex and how this leads to the making of a baby.

A young child might wonder how a baby came to be inside a woman, as an adult might wonder how you get a ship into a bottle.

As part of the gentle flow of information that all parents may have already begun by this age, give very simple, direct information in a matter of fact way. When a child asks a question, parents need to pause and think about what information the child really wants—not how they as an adult might be interpreting the question.

The straightforward information is: 'It takes an egg from a woman and a sperm/seed from a man to make a baby.' This fits all family types, but can be particularly important for children from single parent, or gay or lesbian families, where children will have noticed since about the age of two that they are missing one of the sexes.

It is often important for children from these families to be able to reassure themselves and others that they were made from the same basic ingredients as all human beings.

For heterosexual couples, in which infertility is the reason for the use of egg or sperm donation, language along the following lines can be used: 'Some mommies don't have enough eggs to make a baby and they need another woman to help by giving some of her eggs.'

Or, 'Daddy's sperm couldn't swim fast enough to reach Mommy's egg so we had to go to the doctor and get sperm from a different man.'

The next piece of information, which could be in answer to a question or take place on another occasion entirely, is: 'And that's how you were made.'

At this point, many parents will have their hearts in their mouths, expecting rejection, or long, agonizing and probing questions, but mostly children under five or six carry on with what they were doing, ask what they are having for dinner, or go out and play with the dog. It's all a non-event as far as they are concerned, because what matters to them is the loving relationship they have with their parents.

These are the foundations of children who grow up 'never knowing when they didn't know,' which is recognized by those in family development as the ideal way for children to incorporate donor conception into their sense of who they are.

The story doesn't stop here of course. Parents will need to find ways to keep the subject on the agenda in a gentle and matter of fact way, so that children feel free to ask more evolved questions over time.

Having the conversations does not mean that someday children/ young people won't be curious about their donor, or sad that they are not genetically connected to a much loved parent, or angry that they cannot find further information about their genetic background.

What it does mean is that there will never be a time when donor conception is a shock, or a cause of lack of trust or betrayal in the family, which ideally will always be there to acknowledge feelings and provide the support that young people need in order to make the transition to independent adult life.

Olivia Montuschi, with her husband Walter Merricks, are parents of two donor-conceived young people born in the 1980s. They co-founded with four other families the U.K.-based Donor Conception Network in 1993. Olivia is the author of the "Telling and Talking" booklets for parents of children aged 0 – 7, 8 – 11, 12 – 16 and 17+. These materials are free to download from the website www.DCNetwork.org.

CHAPTER 4

Q&A

WITH WENDY KRAMER

CO-FOUNDER, DONOR SIBLING REGISTRY

Q: What is the most important piece of advice you wish you could convey to all parents of donor-conceived children, based on your experience with thousands of families built by reproductive technology?

The word gamete is used in a clinical setting for the egg or sperm product that is sold to the bank, and then purchased by prospective parents who need it. The term may make it easier for some parents to think of it as simply a cell, or an item of genetic material, and nothing more. But I know very well, from my own teenage son and from the many other offspring I've talked to over the years, that this may not be how they think of it. Many kids do accurately think of the "cell" as one half of their genetic background and heritage. Much more than a clinical product.

So my biggest piece of advice to parents is to let your kids choose for themselves how they define the "gamete" or donor in reference to their life.

My greatest fear is that a child who is told that the donor did nothing more than donate a "cell" grows up unable to express their true thoughts, curiosities and feelings on the matter. I'm no psychologist, but I know this kind of suppression is not healthy—for the child, or for the parent-child relationship.

Again and again, we have heard on the site from donor-conceived adults who have a strong desire to understand this invisible side of themselves. We have heard numerous stories of donor-conceived kids and adults who connect with their donor relatives, either half-siblings or donors, and report it as a profound and meaningful experience.

These people are acknowledging—sometimes even confessing—a genetic bond that is important to them. That's why I urge parents to allow kids to decide for themselves in order to make sure the child doesn't perceive normal curiosity as betrayal, or hurtful to the parent. Please let the discussion and decisions on genetic importance be child-driven, rather than parent-led, over time.

Q: A child who considers the donor important is delivering the kind of situation that most couples want to avoid, right? Isn't that why so many couples decide not to tell their children the truth about their origins? Fear that the donor will replace the non-biological parent, not in day-to-day living, but in emotional connection?

Yes, fear is a main reason couples don't tell. Shame about infertility is another. A large number of men in particular believe it stigmatizes the relationship—or at least their standing in the family—if people know that someone else was required to create that child. This is a very understandable, and common, concern.

But for a parent to relegate their importance in the family as being related to whether they can produce sperm or egg to fertilize an embryo is really, when you think about it, a minor role. I do understand how ego plays a part in these decisions. And it's easy for me to say that it shouldn't matter, since I was able to produce an egg that contributed to my son's birth.

Yet if you ask my son today whether my egg was important to him in terms of my standing as his mother, he would absolutely laugh out loud. We all would, when you look at it that way. And if you ask the people around us whether my egg is the reason I am important in my son's life, they would look at me as if I had lost all sanity.

Our reproductive "goods" have absolutely nothing to do with our role as parents. And to think otherwise is a demeaning position—for ourselves, our partners, and our children.

It might seem contradictory that lack of biological connection means nothing in our parent-child relationship, yet biological connection to the donor might mean so much to our child. But that's exactly the point. A donor is not important to the child in the way we tend to think. As parents, we're off the mark when we think our child wants to find something in the donor that he cannot find in us. Really, we're irrelevant to the story.

Our children want to find connections with donors as extensions of themselves, *not* as extensions of their parents. They *have* parents. What they *don't* have, as fully as they would like, are answers related to their very personal and individualized self-identities. That's something we cannot give them. Only the missing donor can.

Q: Let me press the point a step in another direction, then, as I'm sure many parents are inclined. What, really, can it harm a child to not know the truth of his or her origins? By not telling them they are donor conceived, aren't we really saving them from asking questions that might be difficult to answer?

And why would it be important for them to avoid asking questions about their identity? Every teenager, donor conceived or not, takes that journey. Yes, if they think their father is genetically connected to them, but he is not, it might spare the family some of the questions. But it simply leads to others. A child who doesn't look like his father, and doesn't share some of the same elusive genetic mannerisms, will just as easily wonder why he or she feels unconnected.

Many donor-conceived kids who learn the truth as adults are actually relieved to have an explanation for something they couldn't understand earlier. And then, as adults, they simply have a stronger round of emotions to get through about why their parents didn't respect them enough, or trust them with the information in the first place. Those are even tougher questions to answer, in my opinion.

Q: What, really, is your agenda in developing the Donor Sibling Registry, and in encouraging families to talk about such private matters?

My goal with the discussion group associated with DSR is simply to help educate those of us who made decisions long before we were aware of the true ramifications, so that we can better serve the needs of not only our children, but those to come.

I realize that these discussions can be hot and uncomfortable. It's an emotional area, and we all have different backgrounds and values to respect as we make our own decisions about what is the right thing to do in our families.

But one thing I do recognize is that the donor industry has so far belittled or neglected or forgotten the rights of the children being born. This is a very important debate and until we bring it up for examination, not only among ourselves as donor-conceived families, but in the larger public eye, the industry in the United States will not make any progress.

And I do strongly feel, as did people in the adoption industry before us, that the industry does need to make changes.

Q: Is it the donor industry's job to implement changes, if parents aren't asking for them?

Some parents are asking for them. But as individual voices, or in the occasional media interview. And that's why I'm looking to help them build a stronger, collective voice, so that there is greater impact for the most basic questions we should be talking about.

And yes, most parents do have very different views of what needs to change and what does not. Even our children have different perspectives on what is important to them. We do need to respect the fact that not everyone will agree.

But agreeing to disagree is very different from not having the collective conversation at all. Of course the medical establishment isn't going to lead the discussion. They have no incentive to do so. That's why the kind of conversations that happen on DSR can be perceived as very threatening to them—stirring up debate in an industry that has otherwise been very content to exist on a secretive, private terrain. The thinking among many in the medical establishment that I've talked with is that if it's not broken, why fix it? But of course it IS broken.

> *Many of our kids do suffer from our choices, because we usually aren't thinking them through the way we should. It's that "thinking things through" process that I'm hoping to facilitate.*

I'm not trying to make decisions for families. My goal, really, is to bring up the things I've learned, and enable others to do the same, so that parents can make educated choices.

Q: What frustrates you the most about the choices that some parents are making—decisions that you can try to educate them about, but that are ultimately out of your control?

Without a doubt, it's the shame factor. Unconsciously or not, parents can make it so much more difficult for their children to feel pride about their birth. Obviously our children were wanted. Parents wouldn't go through the steps they do, with something as costly as reproductive technology, if their children were not greatly desired.

Yet a child who doesn't know he was donor-conceived is denied that truth because the parents feel shame, fear, or some other negative emotion. Maybe it doesn't feel that way to the parent. Maybe they genuinely do feel they are protecting their child, perhaps from relatives who might not look favorably on donor conception. Maybe their strong love for the child after birth makes it more difficult to tell the truth, for fear of spoiling the attachment, or adding an artificial ingredient to something that is so powerful a bond.

But in my view, it's never healthy to mislead your child. And it frustrates me that not everyone sees it that way.

In my view, the parent who feels shame about infertility cannot help but project that shame onto the child.

In my view, the couple who feels an imbalance as parents, because one is biologically connected and the other not, have far greater issues to discuss than non-disclosure to the child can cure.

In my view, the parent who holds the perspective that biology is more important than honesty is short-changing the parenting responsibility.

I do have personal experience with several people who are withholding the truth, for various reasons, and it is so foreign to me that I admit I have trouble accepting it. Especially when it relates to my son.

I've had contact with the mother of two of Ryan's half-sisters. The resemblance between her daughters and my son was so strong that she knew after seeing him on TV, without knowing our donor ID number, that they were half-siblings. But she and her husband have no intention of telling their children, who are a few years younger than Ryan, that they were conceived from donor sperm. For Ryan, it's a very sad thing to know that he has half-sisters who quite likely will never know he exists.

Another half-sister, Ryan's age, put a message out on the Internet in search of her donor. She had just been told the truth by her mother, as a teenager, and had a natural curiosity. Someone we know saw the girl's message and sent it to us. Ryan emailed the girl and they enjoyed chatting with each other online, finding many things in common. But after the girl mustered up the courage to tell her mother of the contact, with a note from me in support, the mother took away her cell phone and email account and forbid her to communicate with Ryan.

So once again, Ryan had to work through the anger, frustration and sadness of knowing that there is a half sibling out there that he cannot know. And why? I have been struggling to try to understand this. Trying to understand the threat that Ryan was to that family. Ryan is a good, kind-hearted kid. He would be a positive influence in any half-sibling's life.

This is clearly not about "who" Ryan is, but "what" Ryan is. It hurts me so deeply that my son would be a cause for shame in another family. Such a cause for shame that he is not to be known, and not to be mentioned.

Every day I hear the most amazing stories from DSR members about finding one another. Because of secrecy and shame, this is not so for my own son, and many others. The message that this girl is getting is that somehow the methodology of her conception was shameful. This can be internalized so that a person believes that they are worthy of shame. It's infuriating to me.

As parents of DI kids, don't we owe it to our kids to acknowledge their curiosity and honor their innate right to this curiosity? Why is this so threatening? If the parent is ashamed of having used donor conception, why punish the child with this shame? It's something I simply find frustrating, and hard to understand.

I know not everyone will agree with me. But to me, finding biological family, including half siblings, adds to a child's world—it doesn't subtract. I strongly believe our decisions as parents should be made with the best interests and the rights of the child in mind, not the fears of the adults.

Keeping secrets continues to be the most difficult part of the DI world. At least I know, because DSR is getting hundreds of new members every year who are open to conversation, that more people do recognize that secrets are toxic to families.

Q: Is there anything else you'd like to talk about that we haven't already?

There is a misconception that I am trying to open up donor conception even for those families who want to remain closed. It's true that I do try to "convert" people who are afraid of disclosure or afraid of contact, by demystifying the process for them—and pointing out why I personally think it can add to family life rather than detract from it. And I do share the examples of my son, and others I know who have been affected by donor conception. But it is *not* my intention to expose parents who, for whatever reason, want to keep their families focused solely on the people growing up together under the same roof.

The DSR was formed because my son and I wanted to see if there were others like us, who are openly curious about others who might have come from the same donor, or were at least impacted by donor conception. Since then, thousands have joined us. But I do regularly hear a misconception about the purpose of DSR.

Families and donors who wish to remain anonymous can do so by simply staying off the site. We don't "out" people who don't want their identity known. Certainly we have maintained the privacy of Ryan's other biological family.

There is also a misconception that, since I have raised Ryan alone, and since he is an only child, that I don't understand the dynamics of other families. Of course, I see many types of families everyday, and I do understand why disclosing the truth can be a difficult conversation to start.

I was married when my husband and I agreed to use donor insemination to build our family. The way we conceived was not a factor in the divorce, which happened when Ryan was a baby. I do know the heartache of infertility. And I do know how attractive the option can be of "pretending" that our beloved children were conceived in the most natural way. Yet even if my ex-husband and I had remained married, I know I could never have denied my child the right to the truth about who he is, or curiosity about other biological family that might be out there.

I also know the heartache of not knowing one half of your biological heritage. I have heard the heartache as donor-conceived people find out they have been lied to about their genetic ancestry. The adoption world has come so far in understanding that telling the truth is best and that family secrets can be toxic. I wonder when the prevailing wisdom of donor conception will reach the same conclusions.

VOICES OF OFFSPRING

I call it "going off script." Those uncomfortable, or surprising, or profound moments when your child asks a question or makes a comment that you didn't expect.

Ryan Kramer has given his mother a lot of those moments. At the age of two he asked, "Did my dad die or what?" He was three when he matter-of-factly told her that he had chosen her to be his mother. He was five when he announced that he wanted to learn about electronics. And he was six when he started introducing himself to others with a handshake and a confident, "Hi, I'm Ryan, and I'm a donor baby."

I moderate in-depth discussions with Choice Moms—single women who proactively chose motherhood before finding a partner. I've heard funny and awkward stories about the things our children have said. Such as the preschool boy conceived from an anonymous donor who proudly announced to all of his classmates that he has a father, it's just that his mother doesn't know who he is or where he lives.

My daughter, who was conceived from the same known donor as her younger brother, has heard the stories from a young age about how families are created in different ways. By now she has created several of her own terms for her donor dad. She has drawn a flower, rather than a family tree, to depict the people who are important to her life. She proudly tells new friends, "My mom is a Choice Mom."

It used to be that her questions were simple. But after she turned seven she started to "go off script" with curiosities like: "Who created God?" "But what came before him?"

One night, as we were driving home from a party that had included several new mothers, she asked: "Where do women buy sperm?" I especially stumbled through her next question: "How do men get their sperm out?"

We do prefer that our children stay on script. We want them to think the way we think. We want them to ask only what we can answer—or what we want them to know. But, of course, they are individuals with their own minds. Even at a young age they force us into tough conversations, from why the sky is blue, to where people go after they die, to how sperm finds the egg (and where does it go after that?).

And then, of course, they keep growing. And asking even more sophisticated questions. Some ponder, and don't always ask out loud. As adults, many use the benefit of hindsight to make sense of themselves based on the way they were raised, what they were taught, what rules they were asked to follow.

When they are young, we don't want to be explaining procreation and assisted conception. We don't want them sharing their new knowledge with the neighbors. We don't want them to feel deprived because of choices we have made. We don't want them to notice that we had a bigger say in making biological connections than they do.

In this section, we hear from a teen, a Harvard Law student, and a mother of two. All were conceived from anonymous donor sperm. Their voices remind us that our kids not only come up with their own questions, but independently seek to answer them as well.

There are only two lasting bequests we can hope to give

our children. One is roots; the other wings.

— Hodding Carter

CHAPTER 5

WHY I WANT TO TAKE THE SHAME
OUT OF DONOR CONCEPTION
BY RYAN KRAMER

May 22, 2003 was not an average day for me. In addition to being my 13th birthday, I was scheduled to appear on "The Oprah Winfrey Show," which had been taped several months earlier.

The show was broadcast on the East Coast first. We hadn't yet seen it when the phone started ringing from people who had. Emails started pouring in from viewers who wanted to know how to get their information listed on the Donor Sibling Registry, or to ask general questions about donor insemination. At the time, our website had only a few hundred members, but within a few hours it had started to swell with hundreds of new visitors.

My mom and I took turns overseeing the website, the emails and the phones. In the chaos, my mom glossed over one email she received, which simply asked, "Was that your Ryan on Oprah today?" She replied politely, "yes."

She didn't notice the subject heading: 1058. It referred to my donor's ID number, which had not been mentioned on the show. Troubling.

A few minutes later she received another email from the same person. This time I was fielding the emails, so I saw the message first: "I guess I knew that when I saw him. I gave birth to his two half sisters. They are just as smart and beautiful as he is. I will get back to you more...I am still in shock!"

I had a pile-up of emails that I was trying to fly through. And I hadn't seen the woman's first message, so I was confused when I read this one. But after I read it quickly I froze. I thought to myself, "What is this? Could it be? Nah. Maybe? Yes?"

After reading it over a few more times I yelled at my mom to come look at the screen with me. She knew exactly what it meant. The moment she opened her mouth I heard it in her voice. This was the real deal. I was so excited I wasn't sure what to do. I wrote the woman back desperately trying to verify that she was legit, although I knew she was.

My grandmother had just arrived to watch the show. Together we jumped up and down deliriously, screaming, laughing, crying. The entire reason my mom and I had launched the website was for this moment—when I would find others like myself, who had come from the same donor.

I hopped back on the computer and eagerly wrote the woman a quick note. "I can't believe that after all this time of searching I finally have some closure. This is so exciting. I can't wait for you to write us back with details. This very easily may be the most exciting day of my life. And on top of all of this, it's my thirteenth birthday today! Please write back as soon as humanly possible!!!"

The woman (who we'll call Hannah), replied. Back and forth it went, several times into the evening. She wished me a happy birthday. She told me about her daughters. She said she had secretly compiled information about the donor.

Eventually Mom, Grandma and I drove into town to celebrate my groundbreaking day at a restaurant. On the way, I saw people I knew, stuck my head out the window, and shouted: "I have two half-sisters!" The evening was electric. I could hardly contain myself. I fell asleep ecstatic.

The Next Day

My mom woke me up the next morning with a look on her face.
I knew something was wrong. She proceeded to read me the latest
email from Hannah.

"My children do not know about the donor insemination, and at
this time I have no plans of telling them. They are our children in
every way, and I almost never think about the circumstances of their
conception. I would like to tell Ryan all that I can about the girls
and the information that I have on the donor. The combination of
the 2 short and 2 long profiles gave me enough information that I
feel that if medically necessary I could locate this person. My intent
in contacting you is not to become family members, but to share
information. I know that you will respect that. Saying that, I guess
that I am really not sure what it is that you and Ryan do want."

I didn't really have much of a reaction at first. I lay there quietly,
trying to let it soak in. Eventually I sat up and really thought about it.
It was very disappointing. It had taken years to get this far, and then
it seemed snatched away. And I knew there was nothing I could do
about it.

Ditto

Fast forward three years. I awoke one weekend as normal, staggered
downstairs, poured a bowl of cereal, greeted my mom, and sat
down in front of the television. I heard my mom call me from the
computer. She had that tone in her voice. I immediately knew the
reason she was calling me over.

She showed me an "ad" forwarded to us by one of the registry
members, posted on another site by a 15-year-old girl who was
searching for "Donor 1058."

There was one rogue line: "You see I'm not supposed to search..." It
could have meant a number of things, but at worst I figured it would
be an obstacle that would be easily overcome.

I sat on the information for a day or two, thinking it over, until one afternoon while on campus, I decided to write her an email. It was pretty rudimentary, explaining who I was and how I'd heard of her.

She wrote me back, clearly in shock. It was obvious that she was very nervous, especially about how her mother would react. But she did decide to tell her.

A few days later, I learned that her mom had not taken the news well. She had commandeered her email, cell phone, and myspace account, and confined her to her room. She explained to me via instant messaging that it might take a while for her mom to cool off. But days turned to weeks, and then to months. Hopefully someday she'll be allowed to get to know me.

Dissent Even in the Ranks

I understand that not everyone shares my opinion about the importance of honesty and disclosure. Similarly, I understand that not all donor-conceived children feel the same way about what it means to be a DI kid. When I was 14, in fact, I had to defend myself (and my mother) from the attacks of other donor-conceived kids who didn't think she was doing enough to combat the practice of insemination itself.

As I wrote at 14, and still feel as powerfully today:

> I have never once felt anger or hurt of any sort for being conceived. Certainly I am sometimes curious about my roots, but I am who I am, and knowing my donor wouldn't change that. My mother has not "brainwashed" me, or "tricked" me into being a happy young man. The truth is, not knowing my donor is not something I think about on a day-to-day basis. It's not that I ignore it, but having known it since I was only two years of age has made it a part of my life that I embrace and accept.
>
> You repeatedly say that I "don't know who half of me is." That's absolutely not true. While, indeed I don't know where half of me

came from, I still know what it is. There are parts of me, both physically and emotionally, that I can distinctly pull out of my mother's side. Things about my nose and eyes and hands, and also emotional resemblance. Once I have isolated all of these things, the process of elimination shows me the side I obtained from my donor. So make no mistake, I do see him in myself, in my brown eyes, in my love for math and passion for engineering.

It also was not selfish of my mother to want a child. That's human nature, and if this was the way she (and her ex-husband) were to do it, so be it. I feel that growing up in a one-parent household has brought me closer to my mother, and today we have one of the strongest parent-offspring relationships of anyone I know.

To Be Blunt

I feel sorrow for the donor-conceived kids who may never know their true origins—or worse may discover them in a harmful or damaging way. I pity the weak bond they likely have with their parents as a result of the secrecy. I'm frustrated by the damage that secrets will do to their development. I'm angry at the parents for withholding such important information from their own child, and by proxy creating damage to the child and the bond they have with their child.

In my view, it is foolish and barbaric that secrets like these are still kept.

Seeing so many secrets around me has made me eternally grateful that my mother has raised me in such an open and honest way. Having everything out on the table, and understanding where I came from, has been an important part in defining who I am. The unusually strong bond that I have with her is at least in part a product of the honesty that we've always shared.

While I do feel empathy for parents who are threatened about talking openly about the way their families were built, I feel no compassion for failing to do so.

I understand that this is a subject with very few resources. I understand that it is not as easy for everyone to foresee unexpected consequences as it is for someone like me who has heard them in stories of thousands of DSR members. I understand that parents might disagree about the best approach, or the timing. I understand that any decision a parent makes is thought to be with the child's best interest in mind.

But from my unique perspective, there are clear definitions about the "wrong" way to do things. The "wrong" way is to imply to your kid, directly or indirectly, that there is something shameful about the way they were conceived. The "wrong" way is to withhold (or censure) information about a kid's background so that the parent can feel more comfortable. And the "wrong" way is to treat a donor-conceived child like a secret that should be covered up.

Ryan Kramer finished high school at the age of 14. He is a third-year student in aerospace engineering at the University of Colorado in Boulder. He and his mother co-founded the Donor Sibling Registry in 2000.

CHAPTER 6

OPEN PARENTS, CLOSED SYSTEM

BY REBECCA HAMILTON

I was born in 1977 to two happily married and loving parents. They told me before I could talk that I was conceived with the help of a sperm donor. They were ahead of their time in ignoring the doctor's advice to 'go home, make love, and pretend it's your own child.'

They did everything right by me in dealing with the donor conception issue. I always knew that Dad wasn't my biological father, just as he knew I wasn't his biological daughter. That honesty enabled Dad and I to have a special relationship. He loved me for being my own little human being, and I revelled in being 'Daddy's little girl.'

Dad died when I was nine. The year he died, my mother almost died as well. She was in and out of the hospital after that. Being an only child, I was largely fending for myself from the age of 10. Some might think these facts have something to do with my lifelong quest to find my biological father. But I see it as an entirely separate issue.

What do I know about the man who gave me half of my genes? He donated sperm anonymously in 1976 at National Women's Hospital in Auckland, New Zealand. That's it.

There are many rational reasons why this void would make me frustrated:
  • Half of my ancestry, my ethnicity, is unknown.

• I don't have a full medical history, which puts me at a serious disadvantage for knowing about various genetic predispositions.
• Any future child of mine will be deprived of one-quarter of his or her identity.
• I undoubtedly have half-siblings who are unknown to me.
• Were I still living in New Zealand—a small country by any standard—it is not inconceivable that I could be in a romantic relationship with one of them.

However, these are not the reasons that have led me to waste hours of energy feeling frustrated, depressed and disconnected.

My feelings are difficult to explain to people who take their roots for granted. An adopted person once described the sensation of what is now termed 'genealogical bewilderment' as having to drive through life without a road map. I find it to be an apt description of my situation.

People who know both of their biological parents find it hard to grasp the enormity of what I am missing. Simply having information about the sort of people they are, and what things they are capable of doing, creates a baseline that you don't realize is comforting unless you have to live without it.

I hate that I even have to explain myself like this.

I want to know my biological father just because it's a perfectly natural and human desire to want to look at a man's face and see oneself reflected back in it. I know I look for a reflection of myself in my mother — there's definitely something there in the green eyes, but I'm five inches taller than her, with smaller bones and a different nose. Perhaps if I could find my half-siblings then this urge to see my other traits accounted for would be somewhat alleviated.

People say to me, 'lots of kids don't have a Dad.' In doing so, they completely miss the point at two levels.

1. It's not a 'Dad' I'm after. I had a wonderful Dad who raised

me. I'm not looking for a replacement. Nor, incidentally, is any other donor-conceived person I have ever met.

2. Even people whose parents separated before they were born, or whose fathers died when they were little, usually have something tangible to ground them. Often there are photographs or videotapes. Failing that, there are at least other people who can describe what he was like, how he thought about the world around him, what his mannerisms were.

As you read this, I wonder if you are thinking that I need to stop acting like the glass is half-empty?

With the circumstances that befell my childhood, I ended up without a high school education. Accordingly, I consider myself lucky in the extreme to now be completing my graduate studies at Harvard. I value all the wonderful people in my life, and projects that I have the opportunity to be involved with. And given all this good fortune, I often admonish myself for the frustration and sadness I still feel so deeply.

Yet in a way, the fact that I still feel the loss so strongly—despite having more positive counterweights than any other donor-conceived person I know—only proves the point.

Wanting to understand one's genetic roots is a unique longing that remains no matter how great life is going on other levels.

Of course, the intensity of the loss ebbs and flows. Most of my time is spent focused on other things. But then I'll see a photo in a newspaper of a group of donor-conceived half-siblings who have found each other and will find myself in a flood of tears. Or a friend's parents will come to town to visit and I will look at them together, mesmerized by their similarities. In short, there is nothing that can substitute for what I'm missing. My life is wonderful and fulfilling in the extreme—but the loss is always there and there is nothing anyone can say to make it go away.

People say I should be grateful to the anonymous man who enabled me to exist. Would I rather not be alive?

Prior to starting law school I worked with displaced populations in Sudan. In the process, I interviewed women in camps who were traumatized beyond recognition and yet who still chose life over non-existence. It is human nature to want to survive, and that instinct cannot be taken as an indication of contentment with the conditions in which one is living. Donor-conceived people are the only group our society places this existential debt upon. If I were conceived through rape, would people expect me to be grateful to the rapist?

People tell me that I am special because my parents wanted me so much.

Lots of children are wanted. Feeling wanted is not a substitute for having access to your identity.

People tell me that perhaps if I met my biological father I wouldn't like him anyway and that many people who know their fathers wish they didn't.

Give me that option—to decide if I like him.

During college, I couldn't accept the sheer helplessness of my situation. Lines of inquiry through doctors and the hospital had been fruitless. However, I felt strongly that a donor who agreed to be anonymous more than 20 years ago might have a different opinion today.

I got some confirmation of this belief after speaking with a researcher at the University of Auckland, Dr. Vivienne Adair. She had done a study of men who had been donors under a contract of anonymity. A full 98 percent of them said they were happy to provide non-identifying information if their biological children wanted it. Many also said they were willing to provide identifying information, and expressed an interest in meeting 'offspring.'

If a donor choses to remain anonymous that's one thing, but I wanted to at least give my donor the option. Since there were no records of donors for me to access, I decided the only way to give him this option was to use the media. That decision led me to make a documentary about my search, "Are You My Father?" It screened nationally in New Zealand in 2001, and was a catalyst for legislative changes that followed.

What I Learned From My Documentary

In 18 months of filming, I did DNA tests with six donors. None of them were my biological father. But I came out of the process having met six men who are the biological fathers of New Zealand children they have never met.

In that anxious period when you wait for DNA results, there are inevitable 'what if?' questions. All of the men I tested were clear that they did not want to intrude on my life. Although they were genuinely curious about whether I might be their daughter, their agreement to DNA testing was driven by my need to know, not theirs.

The new legislation ensures that all donors must provide identifying information that is centrally recorded and available to donor-conceived children after they reach 18 years of age. So although I didn't find my donor, there is some consolation in knowing that from 2005 onwards, no child born through donor conception in New Zealand will be in the same position that I am.

After the documentary screened, I got a lot of emails from parents saying they'd like to be truthful with their kids, they just didn't quite know how to start explaining it.

I've talked with many biological and non-biological parents, as well as donor-conceived people. Here are some of the things I've learned:

- **It's important to start early.** There is now plenty of literature from both the adoption and donor-conception areas to suggest that kids sense that something about their birth is "off." Donor-conceived people who don't learn the truth until they are adults often report that they grew up imagining that their mother had an extra-marital affair, or that they were adopted. Finding out that they are donor-conceived is often a confirmation of intuitions they already had. By contrast, being told the truth from the beginning allows the whole thing to feel 'normal' and matter-of-fact. "My name's Rebecca, my cat's called Smudge, a donor helped make me, and school holidays start tomorrow."

• **Even if you aren't sure how to define "family," have faith that your children know the difference between "real" and "biological."** It can be terrifying for the non-biological parent to think about the child having contact with the donor. They imagine phrases like "you're not my real Dad," or fear the child will be confused about who is the parent. But when you are the one changing the diapers, driving to the sports practice, going over homework, there is no doubt who the parent is. Children know their parents are the people who raise them. When donor-conceived people search out their biological roots, it is not to find 'replacement' parents, it is to complete their own identities.

• **Telling the truth from the outset gives parents great freedom from the burden of secrecy.** Secrets invariably get discovered — accidentally, purposefully, unconsciously. Too often I've spoken to people who found out late, and more than learning that their Dad isn't who they thought he was (most of them had kind of guessed as much already), the far greater problem is 'how could they lie to me about something so fundamental for so many years?' That's a hard foundation to rebuild any relationship on.

My Three Core Beliefs

1. It is simply wrong to create human beings with the intent that they will not be able to access their genetic information.

To be sure, there are people born into circumstances that prevent them from accessing both genetic parents—for instance, people born as the result of a one night stand, or even rape. However that is not the same thing as having families and clinics legally create human beings with the a priori intention of keeping information from them.

In an ideal world, everyone would have access to family history. Of course, it's not an ideal world and there are some situations we don't have control over, but reproductive technology is not one of them.

2. Openness is not a substitute for open-identity.

The openness of my parents in talking with me about being donor conceived is, I believe, a model for anyone considering donor conception. Since my donor search began, my mother has been nothing but supportive. However, my story shows that even the most sensitive and respectful handling of the issue cannot substitute for, or alleviate, the fundamental urge to know one's biological parents.

Not every child will grow up into a teenager or adult who wants to know their donor. However, when a child is conceived there is absolutely no way of predicting whether he or she will turn out to be one of those children who isn't interested, or one of those children who finds it to be an all-consuming obsession and cause of depression, or anywhere between these extremes. I believe prospective parents should only use identifiable donors. This is the only way they can be sure to have options covered for their child, whose best interests they should have at heart.

Having an identifiable donor does not mean a child is required to meet the donor. It simply means that if your child does have a strong desire to see the face of the person who gave them half their genes— or ask questions of him or her—you haven't foreclosed that option.

3. Access to reproductive technology is not more important than access to identity.

The infertility industry is whipping up a frenzy (especially in the U.K. at the moment) by arguing that requiring donors to be identifiable will lead to a reduction in donors, and that this will harm infertile people.

Experience from countries that have moved to identifiable-only donors shows that there is an initial drop-off in numbers, but the numbers climb back up again with a different kind of donor. Rather than having college students donating sperm for money with no real concept of the implications, you instead see that donors are older, typically married men, who already have healthy children of their own. They understand the gift of children, and that a sense of genetic continuity is important to most human beings.

However, even if there was a drop-off of donors, I do not see this as a reason to continue a system of anonymity. If one believes, as I do, that the use of anonymous donors is wrong, then the practice does not become 'right' merely because it is more available.

People say that a reduction in the donor pool will harm infertile people who want the chance to raise a child. This argument takes us to the heart of the matter. If raising a child is the only issue, then adopted children fit the bill equally well. Prospective parents typically choose donor conception over adoption because they prefer to raise a biologically related child.

> *If the desire for a biological connection is strong enough to make adults choose donor conception over adoption, then it is the ultimate double standard to imagine that the desire for a biological connection will not be felt just as strongly by the donor-conceived person that results.*

I believe our thinking on this issue has been distorted by a medical model that sees infertility as a problem to which the creation of a baby is the solution. People need to understand that donor-conception does not create a 'baby.' It creates a human being who is forced to live with the lifelong consequences of choices made by the adults involved in their creation.

Rebecca Hamilton is a Knox Fellow at Harvard Law School and the John F. Kennedy School of Government. She will complete a joint JD and Master of Public Policy in 2007.

CHAPTER 7

WHEN THE
CHILDREN GROW UP

BY KAREN,
A DONOR-CONCEIVED WOMAN AND MOTHER

At the age of 18, after the death of my father, my mother told me that I was donor conceived. That was more than 20 years ago.

Although I have had time to reflect, explore, research and embrace the nature of my conception as part of my personal narrative, I still wrestle as a grown adult with the issues I share with many of the donor conceived, who inevitably struggle to find comfort in the unknown parts of their genetic identity.

First, my background. I am the only child of parents who tried eight years to conceive before turning to infertility specialists. It was determined that a childhood illness suffered by my father rendered him infertile. They were devastated. Although they did consider adoption, they believed that extended family might have difficulty accepting an adopted child as one of their own. My mother found a local doctor who was willing to help her conceive through the use of an anonymous donor. I was born in upstate New York in 1966.

As a young adult, I attended college in Boston, then moved to Manhattan to work in advertising. I live in the Northeast with my husband, and am a stay-at-home mother to two school-aged children.

In keeping with the times, my parents were advised to keep the origins of my birth confidential, and to pretend that the insemination never happened. But the secret was a terrible burden on them. They had no outlets, other than each other, and felt trapped and alone in keeping this secret. My mother confessed to me that it was an underlying source of tension within their marriage.

It also had created an inequality in their parenting relationship with me, which I detected in innumerable ways—through subtle clues, innuendos and vague responses that human nature couldn't disguise.

For example, whenever I attempted to find similarities with my Dad and his side of the family—which I brought up quite a few times— my parents would smile, avert their eyes, and change the subject.

My mother intensely researched her family's genealogy. When I expressed interest in my paternal family history, I was given the impression that it wasn't significant.

My mother revealed the truth after my father passed away from cancer. The emotions I felt — and continue to feel — are difficult to describe.

Mixed Emotions

I was being told that my biological father was a nameless, faceless person. All the experiences that I thought I understood about my identity, I began to second guess. I was shocked, but it answered so many unspoken questions.

At the same time, I felt illegitimate, ashamed, unrecognized and abandoned by my biological father. This might sound melodramatic to people who haven't been donor conceived, but quite honestly, the questions I pondered in my early adult years included: Why wouldn't he want to know me or be a part of my life? Didn't this mean I was a shameful secret, not only in my own family, but in my biological father's family as well? When I saw people I resembled I wondered, is that Him? Could that be my half-sister or brother?

I knew I could never ask these questions out loud. They would sound absurd. In hindsight, I can see that my self esteem was faltering, but I never shared my feelings with anyone.

Yet I was grateful to know this truth about myself. My mother knew that it would create as many questions as it answered, but she respected and trusted my ability to decide what this meant to me.

She had given me the knowledge I needed to grow as a person. The disclosure marked the beginning of my journey in search for my full identity and, ultimately, allowed me to find greater meaning and understanding.

What I Did With the Information

After the disclosure, I felt alone but never angry. I was too busy putting all the pieces of the rest of my puzzle together. I would quiz my mother occasionally about the particulars of my conception. I was apprehensive about believing the story, but I couldn't imagine that she would have made it up.

Nonetheless, I kept asking, looking for inconsistencies in her story. Did she know for sure daddy was infertile? Why did they decide to do it? Why didn't they adopt? Who was the doctor? How was it done? How many times? Most importantly, who is my biological father?

She could answer all the questions but the last one. The only thing she could tell me about Him was the information that her doctor had given her.

In the 1960's, the donor was a doctor in the same area that we lived, of Northern European heritage, with a family 'of his own.' Other than that, it was up to my imagination.

My imagination left me with so many more questions and revelations. I might have more grandparents, aunts, uncles, and cousins. I might even have siblings! I was excited. I couldn't wait to find these people and introduce myself. We shared a biological connection. We were family! I was sure they'd want to meet me.

My mother, who loved me more than anyone, realized that the information she had to offer was not enough for me. She contacted the doctor who inseminated her and he agreed to speak with me on the telephone.

Closed Doors

I was so nervous when the time came that I could barely speak. I didn't know how to organize all my questions. My voice was quivering. My mind went blank. He simply repeated to me what he had already told my mother. Although he was not forthcoming, as I stumbled through my questions I managed to find out that the donors he used all shared German ancestry and had no family history of inheritable diseases.

He suggested that my dad might still, in fact, be my biological father. I didn't question it. We said goodbye. I hung up the phone and cried for my two lost fathers.

I swallowed my emotions and clung to the doctor's suggestion that my Dad might still be my biological father, but intuitively I knew it wasn't so.

Time has passed quickly, as well as my hope for resolution. I am now married with children and it has become clear that the repercussions of my biological father's anonymity have extended far beyond my own personal enigmas. Our children's full genetic identities, heritage, ancestry, connections and family medical histories have been compromised as well. They are prohibited from knowing who their genetic cousins are, which brings the risk of accidental consanguinity. But regrettably the door is closed. I will never know for certain who my biological father is and I cannot take my search any further.

Belonging

Thankfully, my Dad—the man who agreed to my conception and unselfishly raised me as his own—was a beautiful person and I would never have attempted to replace him.

I wish I could have told my Dad that it doesn't matter whether he and I were biologically connected, that I could not have loved him more if he were my own genetic father.

In fact, knowing the full truth, and the unacknowledged personal sacrifices that my Dad made for the sake of his family, has only added to my adoration.

After all, I am the product of my parents' union. I was conceived of their love and intentionally brought into this world because of their commitment and desire for a child. In our particular situation, any relationship with the donor would have created further complexities and tensions within both of our families.

What Bothers Me the Most?

We know how difficult it can be to blend families, from the experiences of children (and adults) of divorce. But in my case, it was decided by the loved ones in my life, as directed by the professional advice of the era, that I should not know, for at least the first 18 years of my life, the existence of another person who enabled me to be.

Even after I was told the true nature of my conception I was encouraged to consider him as nothing more than a source of some of my DNA, a "mere sperm donor." This was considered to be in all of our best interests.

Yet no one discussed the psychological burden involved in keeping the secret. No one considered how my Dad might feel raising a child conceived by his wife and another (albeit unknown) man. No one anticipated that I might someday learn the truth and have to deal with all the years of unknowing. No one predicted how I would feel about the truth of my origins. And no one speculated about how important this missing piece would be to my children and me.

Our forebears are a part of us in a very deep and profound way. It is my strong view that it is misleading and dehumanizing to refer to my disconnected genetic father—my children's genetic grandfather—as nothing more than a mere "donor."

I feel that to intentionally reduce a genetic parent to nothing more than a source of sperm or egg demeans our need for genetic identity, heritage, ancestry and connections.

> *Especially as an adult, with children of my own, I do not like to be told how I should feel, or what I should call, the person who is one-half of my genetic make-up.*

In my situation, I understand why this well intentioned "service" was contingent on anonymity. Although that does not make it any less painful to feel that the person who is a permanent part of my family's bloodline does not know, is socially prohibited from, or is disinterested in knowing anything about us or being a part of our lives.

Even now, more than 20 years after disclosure, my origin story continues to carry with it a stigma of illegitimacy. I was never a consenting party to the anonymity agreement yet my search for truth is still considered by some as something to be ashamed of and something I should be fearful of sharing.

Perhaps my deepest regret is that my Dad felt he had to hold this secret to his death in order to protect me.

What If We Were Infertile?

I ask myself often, if my husband was infertile, what would we do? I always imagined myself as a mother. I knew that I wanted to have children 'of my own' someday. I wanted to have babies that shared my biology and pour myself into their nurturing and well being. I wanted to feel them kicking inside of me, inhale them and know that they were 'mine.' This must be a primal instinct.

The pain of infertility must be overwhelming. My mother must have had this same need...instinct....that I do. She married a man that she loved more than anything in her world. He adored her and she him.

But the two of them could not physically produce the one thing she instinctually wanted—a baby of 'their own.'

I wonder if men have the same need and instinct as women do? I wonder how my Dad felt when he found out that the reason they hadn't conceived was because he couldn't produce sperm. They must have mourned deeply for the children they could not create together.

He loved my mother immensely and would have done anything for her. Together, they found a doctor who was willing to do something that no one else in the area was willing or pioneering enough to do—artificial insemination by anonymous sperm.

The advice of the day was secrecy, so that everyone, including the child, would accept each other without prejudice or discrimination.

So I question again, what would we do? If I wasn't donor conceived myself, and didn't have the benefit of knowing how this has affected my parents and me, my husband and I might do the most convenient thing: buy or borrow another man's sperm.

But I know from my personal experience how difficult this choice is, not only for the child, but for the parents, the donor, the donor's extended social family. Even open donations might create and/or lead to conflicts of loyalty, identity and belonging. Although the inability to have a genetic child of my own would create deep sadness, I know in my heart that donor conception is just not something that we could do.

SECTION THREE

VOICES OF REFORM

In Fall 2006, I was asked to speak to a group of sperm bank directors about what reform might be needed in their industry, based on my conversations with Choice Moms who make up one-third to one-half of their client base, as well as with other people represented in this book.

My primary suggestions were to create a national registry for anonymously tracking births and medical histories for each donor, and to develop an awareness campaign for donors and recipients at the start of the process—when donating or purchasing sperm.

The jury is still out on what the directors of the roughly 22 major U.S. sperm banks will do differently. But it is clear that a few of them are listening to the concerns expressed by parents and offspring—sometimes because of the public relations headaches that result from complaints voiced in the media—and are grappling with what their ethical, legal and social responsibilities should be.

For this section, we hear from a parent, a donor-conceived adult, and a donor about their wish list of industry changes. They do not speak for everyone. But they are articulate, impassioned individuals—with backgrounds we've explored elsewhere in this book—with remarkably clear suggestions for how they believe the industry could be improved going forward, based on what we've learned from the past.

My Top Five Wish List of
Changes for the Industry
By Wendy Kramer

Although I know everyone needs to make the choices that are right for them, there are so many things I wish we were doing differently as collective participants in the donor conception industry—parents, donors, doctors, sperm banks.

#1: The infertility industry needs to move forward with the best interests of the children being born in mind.

This is what drives everything for me, and what I will push to become the mantra of everyone involved in the industry: How can we best serve the needs of the child being born?

Not the best interests of making money. Not the best interests of donors who want to leave their genetic material at the door and not have some communication with the children that result. Not the best interests of recipients (like me) who simply want to have a baby.

Let's start making decisions and setting policy with the best interests of the children in mind. Let's start talking openly about questions such as: Is it acceptable to bring a child into the world who does not know half of their genetic background? Can we ethically allow recipients to withhold the fact from their children that an outside party was largely responsible for their conception? If we do this, whose needs are we serving?

#2: Sperm banks need to be uniformly held responsible for keeping accurate records.

It's been reported that only 40 percent of women report their live births to sperm banks. Some banks make this a stronger priority and have a much higher reporting record; many others do not. How can this be remedied?

Without accurate records, there is no way of knowing how many offspring come from the same donor. Without accurate records, there is no way of contacting families that share the same donor if offspring end up sharing genetic diseases. Without accurate records, there is no reason for a donor to report a later history of heart disease or breast cancer or depression in his/her family, because there is no way of informing offspring.

Since banks also share donated gametes with other banks as well (why they do this, I'm not sure, but we know from the packaging information that this is so), it's important to know how many kids are coming from the same donor, even if it's from different banks.

As the point of purchase, sperm banks are the best and most efficient source of keeping track of this information.

#3: Track donors and their medical histories.

This goes hand-in-hand with point #2. Without a better system of record-keeping for all institutions involved in donor conception, there is no way we can best serve the interests of the children—and their children.

I strongly urge sperm banks to mandate, as a condition of becoming accepted as a donor, that they need to report annually any changes in medical history. If a donor is willing to undergo numerous screens and blood tests, abstain from sex, and go behind closed doors on a regular basis to provide semen for cash, they certainly should be expected to accurately and proactively provide up-to-date medical histories for the offspring that result.

With this comes another important factor in the triad. As communication between donors and parents and offspring improves, better legal protection must be implemented at a federal level so that donors everywhere don't have to fear child support lawsuits and so that parents everywhere don't have to fear child custody battles.

#4: Mandate counseling for recipients and donors.

Families and donors should not be blindsided five, ten and 15 years later by the fact that kids are proving to be very curious and wanting answers. We know from the past two decades that this is the case.

Sperm banks and clinics—again, as the point of "purchase"—need to recommend a list of fertility counselors for any recipient looking for donor conception service. Just as adoption agencies require prospective parents to undergo a home study, so that issues are explored that the parent might not have considered in order to ensure that a child is being brought into a well-prepared environment in which his/her best interests will be served.

Similarly, at the informational meeting that every sperm bank has with prospective donors—who sometimes are lured there with the promise of movie tickets and free food and the opportunity to earn hundreds of dollars each month to "do what you'd be doing anyway"—there should be a mental health counselor to also talk about the long-term implications of this choice. Such as:

• Raising the kinds of questions kids will want to be able to ask him, anonymously or in an open-identity situation.
• Stipulating the need to regularly update the bank on medical history so that real families with real kids can be informed over time.
• Pointing out that misinformation on medical history forms today, in order to be accepted as a donor, will affect real lives.

#5: Mandatory disclosure.

The reform I've suggested so far is easy. After all, why wouldn't we want to keep confidential records of offspring and donors, in case of emergencies. And why wouldn't we want to let newcomers know what we already know from previous generations about how donor conception affects parents, donors and offspring?

On the other hand, mandatory disclosure of donor conception to children treads on the kind of "entering the family home" territory we tend to get nervous about. It's controversial to suggest that we must require parents to do anything. But again, for me, it comes down to the integrity and mental health of the environment for the child. How can we overlook a person's inherent right to know where they came from? Their ancestry? Their family history?

Don't we know as a society that family secrets are toxic? Haven't we learned this from walking in the footsteps of the adoption world? I have heard from so many adult donor conceived who tell of finding out the truth later in life—often after years of suspecting something was wrong about them—and feeling deceived and betrayed.

The reproductive industry needs to reshape itself so that it honors a child's curiosity and right to know their genetic heritage, rather than the archaic notion that if conception does not occur in the "normal" way there is something shameful and secretive that the child must be protected from. Why would we want donor conception to remain some dirty little secret? Why wouldn't we want our kids to know the great lengths we went in order to bring them into our lives?

After all, whose secrets are we keeping?

There is a difference between privacy and secrecy. There is a way to honor everyone's needs.

Parents and donors must be forewarned that kids have the right to know certain things. It is, after all, the kids who are affected most by the decisions we make today.

ABOLISH ANONYMITY,
EVEN IF IT DOESN'T SOLVE EVERYTHING

BY KAREN,
A DONOR-CONCEIVED WOMEN AND MOTHER

The emotional issues of people born of donor conception are not unlike those of adoptees. In fact, assisted reproduction has been recognized as a form of adoption, and incorporated into the American Adoption Congress mission statement: Through education and advocacy, the AAC promotes honesty, openness and respect for family connections in adoption, foster care and assisted reproduction.

Many proponents of assisted reproduction argue that we must learn to accept the emotional complexities of our birth as a condition of our existence and be grateful for what we have. This is true. We do not want to become consumed by our frustrations.

But all too often those of us who express feelings of loss or anger over having been born from assisted reproduction are considered selfish or ungrateful. We are cautioned that anything less than gratitude would hurt our parents and would be disrespectful to others who choose to form a family using these methods. Existential debt serves as a strong suppressant for many of our voices and concerns.

Each individual's circumstances and feelings will be unique. Several parents of donor-conceived children have stated in various online forums and in the media that their children have no interest in knowing who their donors are. They point out that the well-adjusted and content donor-conceived people rarely speak up because it holds no interest for them.

And, of course, there are many people born from anonymous donors who are unaware of the nature of their conception. Of the ones who know, it is not surprising that some might not care, or say they are happy they were conceived under these circumstances. Some might not have strong feelings at the moment but may change over time. Others might find it too difficult to explore, or fear what they will find if they do. Some might wish they had never been told. Others might only want medical information, perhaps a picture. Some might want to meet half siblings or speak to their donors. Some might simply want them to know who they are. But for some, including myself, having a name, medical information, or being able to meet once or occasionally will still leave a void. Some of us with disenfranchised grief long for meaningful human connection with our genetic fathers.[1]

I relate to, for example, the views of Wendy Rowney, a Canadian adoptee who advocates in the Toronto adoption community.[2] She wrote:

> *Many people will argue that this pain will disappear if we can only guarantee that adoptees and donor-conceived people can learn of their roots. There is no doubt that access to this information does help, but I believe that the pain stems from the dislocation we feel. Where do we truly belong? Nowhere. We find love in our families, but we can see that we are different. We may be lucky enough to find love in our [birth] families, but we were missing for so many years that we often don't truly belong there either. We are also coming to terms with the fact that our (genetic) parents…chose instead to give us away. In doing so, they also gave away our heritage, our ethnicity and our ancestry. These are not unimportant things. They matter. We have to mourn these losses. Knowing the*

name of our (genetic) parent(s) doesn't make the pain go away and so I would argue that it is adoption/donation itself that causes this pain; it is not solely the absence of knowledge.

There is very little research that studies the experience and perspective of donor-conceived adults. Bill Cordray, a donor-conceived adult from the United States who has spoken and written about DI issues for nearly 20 years, has been compiling a Survey on the Attitudes of Donor Conceived People about Secrecy, Disclosure and Access to Information.[3] To date he has had 91 donor-conceived adult respondents, ages ranging from 18-59.

He began the survey in 1999 as part of a presentation he had made at the 11th World Conference on IVF in Sydney, Australia. Participants were recruited from support groups and the Internet. He has since expanded on this survey to include many of the DI adults he has since met. The DI adults in his study come from the U.S., the U.K., Canada, Australia, New Zealand and Japan.

The results are fascinating but not surprising. In particular:
- 100% feel the right to know the donor's medical history
- 97% believe that children born from donors should be told
- 81% want to know the donor's identity
- 81% want to contact the donor
- 77% want to meet the donor and half-siblings
- 74% believe knowing as young as possible is best
- 58% of participant's parents are divorced

Out of the divorced families:
- 69% were told after their parents divorced
- 45% felt the secret played a role in their parents' divorce

Where do we go from here?

We know that genetic relation does not guarantee ideal parenting or family environment. But we also know that genetic connections are important anchoring points for an individual. Have we not learned from the vast research and studies on the ramifications of kinship separation, or "genealogical bewilderment," in the adoptive experience?

Why should an adult's want for a child take precedence over a person's need for meaningful connection with their full genetic identity, heritage and kin?

If nothing else, our country desperately needs to find a way to regulate the reproductive technologies industry to provide for the needs of the children as well as the parents. The United Nations Convention on the Rights of the Child, sanctioned by all 190 members of the United Nations except the United States and Somalia, acknowledges, in articles 7 and 8, the child's right to know and be cared for by his or her parents and the right of the child to preserve his or her identity, including nationality, name and family relations as recognized by law without unlawful interference.

Moving forward, donor anonymity needs to be addressed. Even though I recognize the complications it can bring to family life when contact with a donor is made in later years, as an adult I strongly believe it is my right to negotiate those connections.

1. I believe the United States should follow in the footsteps of the Netherlands, Germany, Italy, Sweden, Norway, Switzerland, Austria, England and Finland, which have banned the anonymous buying and selling of human sperm and eggs.

2. Limits need to be set on the number of offspring sired per donor. Every child born from these services need to be accounted for and clearly identified.

3. Payment for sperm, eggs and surrogates should be limited to actual expenses incurred.

4. The practice needs to work towards openness and honesty, identifying both the social parents as well as genetic parents on

birth certificates.

Reproductive technologies are here to stay, for better or for worse, but it desperately needs regulation to protect the interests of the people born from it who have no voice and no choice.

ENDNOTES

[1] Kenneth Doka, editor of the book *Disenfranchised Grief: Recognizing Hidden Sorrow*, defines this type of grief as emotion that is connected with a loss that cannot be openly acknowledged, publicly mourned or socially supported. He says that in many cases of disenfranchised grief, the relationship is not recognized, the loss is not recognized, or the griever is not recognized.

Joanna Rose, a donor-conceived woman who has played an active role in the abolishment of donor anonymity in the United Kingdom, first wrote about this grief as it applies to the donor conceived in a paper titled, *From a 'bundle of joy' to a person with sorrow: Disenfranchised grief for the donor-conceived adult* (Queensland University of Technology Applied Ethics Seminar Series, 2001).

[2] Excerpted with Rowney's permission from a Yahoo discussion group, Donor Misconception.

[3] Survey results shared with permission by Bill Cordray.

MORE HIGHLY SCREENED DONORS, UNLIMITED OFFSPRING

BY KIRK MAXEY

A few years ago, if you did a Google search on my name, you could retrieve several pages of references to scientific papers I had written, to my position in the Lipid Maps consortium, and to things that I had worked hard to achieve. Now, if you do that same search, you get things like ABC Nightline's "Confessions of a Sperm Donor."

I never wanted to be sensationalized for this activity, and it's frustrating to be defined by the media as needing a "confessional." Yet it is essential to me that I get involved. I am deeply suspicious of the sperm banking industry, and believe some of them have used the shield of anonymity to cover fraudulent practices. The sperm bank where I donated for more than a decade resisted providing me even with my own donor ID number. All of this secretive activity builds a sense of shame around the entire process, which seems quite unnecessary.

I strongly believe that regulatory guidelines need to be enacted to mandate what information must be collected, what must be disclosed, and what contact information must be kept on an ongoing basis. Those in the medical establishment who refuse to look up records that would help connect donors and siblings who want to make contact are not breaking laws, but I believe they are abusing their position of trust as the keepers of their clients' and donors' genetic and medical histories.

Focusing on Genetic Issues

Many prospective parents seeking infertility treatment are concerned about the health of children conceived from reproductive technology. They distrust the artificial nature of the procedure, and worry that it will cause defects in their child. But as a former donor who specializes in biomedical research and development, I know that the freezing, thawing, and other artificial steps used in donor sperm insemination have been documented extensively in both humans and animals to have no effect on the health of the offspring.

As a secondary concern, some parents also worry about the genetic pedigree of the donor. In this instance, however, they generally concede that their own pedigree is not likely to be perfect, and they seem willing to accept the normal risk that everyone has that a defect will come from either of the biological parents.

And in fact, in the general population, there are thousands of couples who know full well that they are carriers of devastating diseases, yet they choose to conceive in the hope that nature's roll of the dice will land in their favor. Roughly 25 percent of the time they lose, and a "defective" child is born.

I do think, however, that there is a reason that genetic health of a sperm donor can and should be held to a higher standard than the average population.

A Brief History of Sperm Insemination

Before discussing specific areas of health concern, it is important to note how donor insemination itself has changed over time. The entire field has been shrouded in secrecy. There are no records to indicate how rapidly DI grew as an accepted regimen for childless couples, but it is clear that during the first few decades DI was not a big business.

The patients were virtually all married heterosexual couples. The donors during this early era were simply family members of the couple, colleagues of the doctor, or (unethically) the doctor himself. Thus, the donors were not selected for above average height or education, as they are today, and so are probably also representative of the population at large.

Semen was used fresh and without any testing or freezing, so there is very little to distinguish early DI from normal conception, except for the unconventional genetic architecture between the donor, the offspring and the parents. More than 90 percent of these couples never told anyone, including the child, that they used DI.

In the face of this information vacuum, it is very unlikely that the period between 1940 and 1980 can ever be properly studied.

Since then, however, it has been an entirely different era for donor insemination. Heterosexual couples experiencing male infertility have fallen into the minority in some places. Single women choosing to become mothers and lesbian couples wishing to have children have become a much greater part of the population of DI clients. In both cases, talking to the child openly about origins—including some amount of information about the donor—has become commonplace.

Perhaps the only consistent demographic factor connecting the two eras is that DI has remained overwhelmingly Caucasian.

The collection and marketing of donor semen also has changed dramatically. Today it has become a big business, served by roughly 20 sperm banking corporations, rather than hundreds of small fertility clinics typically connected to medical schools.

Regulation of infectious disease such as HIV has made all donor semen subject to a unique freezing process, to enable a six-month quarantine for testing purposes. Roughly 10% of men produce semen of adequate number and viability to overcome the freezing process in a reliable way, dramatically reducing the total number of potential semen donors.

At the same time, sperm banks sharply increased the compensation provided to donors, introducing commercial factors into the recruitment and qualification of donors.

The Demographics of Donor Conception

On the female side of the equation, the age of the mothers trying to conceive through DI is well above the population average, which itself has moved upward as couples and single women have delayed starting their families until the third decade of life. Many are conceiving in their forties, making them far from ideal candidates for conception and pregnancy in general. Careful genetic counseling and prenatal screening can help improve the chances that these mothers will give birth to a healthy baby.

Sperm donors face two screens: one for the absolute quantity and physical vigor of their spermatozoa, both fresh and after being frozen and re-thawed. Secondly, the donors are questioned extensively about their own health and the health of family members.

In my opinion, however, this latter test has been badly compromised during the last decade by the escalating compensation being paid to the donor. Donor compensation remains the largest confounding factor that may compromise donor quality. Prospective applicants now have an economic incentive to "polish" their family medical histories, leaving out sick or disabled relatives and even omitting diseases from their own medical pedigrees. This deceit enables them to have access to substantial compensation, which in many cases can be several hundred dollars per week.

It is unlikely that deceitful donors represent more than a small minority of the total donor pool, but their presence can still compromise the overall safety of donor semen.

The genetic and fertility biases present in modern DI represent a curious mix. The women tend to be of above average intelligence, age, and socioeconomic status. As already mentioned, they are overwhelmingly Caucasian. They bring genetic risks typical of North Europeans, such as Tay Sachs disease, cystic fibrosis, and hemochromatosis. Their risk of Downs syndrome is elevated in conjunction with their maternal age. If there are genetic factors associated with lesbianism, they are overrepresented in the client population, as are factors associated with single mothers who are independent and self-sufficient.

On the male side, the sperm banks provide the type of donors that women seem prone to select. This has slanted the donor pool heavily in favor of increased height and advanced education. The application of genetic screening tests and donor family medical questionnaires should be acting to reduce the overall frequency of defective genes in this population, although the degree to which this has happened cannot be quantified.

In theory, DI parents have purchased semen that is pre-qualified to have a lower risk of certain genetic diseases than the general population.

In practice, of course, DI parents don't always get "perfect" children. Genetic diseases are passed along—sometimes mutations from a parent's untested DNA, sometimes anamolies in DNA from the donor that were not tested.

An Overseas Example of the Issues

In February 2002, doctors at a Dutch hospital sent letters to 13 families in the Netherlands who had used a particular semen donor. For three years, these doctors had known that the donor was a carrier of a genetic disorder called ADCA, and that the 18 children he had fathered in these families had a 50 percent chance of having inherited the disease from him. If so, the ADCA gene they were carrying would cause them to stumble, slur their speech, become demented, and die, with these symptoms beginning in their mid thirties to mid forties.

Two years later, and in part as a response to this scandal, the Dutch parliament passed a law limiting the number of live births permitted to any sperm donor to 10.

If there is a lesson to be drawn from the ADCA incident, it may be summarized by saying this, "There is no risk-free semen."

Why the U.S. Industry Needs Reform

For me, the issue becomes problematic when sperm banks, who have access to donor records, hold privacy of the donor (including mine) and other families in greater esteem than the rights of parents and offspring to learn as much as they can about any genetic issues.

In my view, privacy of willing participants in reproductive technology is one matter that is trumped when access to medical information is needed. I think all participants in the process should be made aware of that at the start—as well as after the fact, when issues arise.

The major problem I have with the industry today is that the commercial sperm bank that buys and sells the semen—and the potential defendant in any civil action—is the go-between that is responsible for receiving information about defects, responding to this information, and making any necessary investigations. It is a classic conflict of interest.

What Are the Risks?

Genetic risk is a very difficult thing to measure. Each of us has, within our own brain, a subtle calculus for estimating the risks of defects in the people that we might choose to mate with. We actively reject people with skin discolorations, asymmetrical eyes, ears or other features, and those with body weights outside a fairly narrow range. On the behavioral side, we reject those who seem antisocial, while favoring those who seem clever, witty, engaging, and empathetic. Without bringing an ounce of science to the table, each of us has intuitive mechanisms for detecting both the shallow and the deep ends of the gene pool.

However, most genetic disease is both complex and invisible. Take for example, the gene BRCA1 that predisposes one to increased risk of certain cancers. There is no overt way to spot someone with a defective BRCA1 gene. There are also many ways in which the gene can be defective—some severe, and some not. Some mutations involve just one base in the DNA sequence—a single nucleotide polymorphism (or SNP). That would be analogous to having one single misspelled word in this book.

Yet there are *dozens* of different SNPs just in the BCRA1 gene. Imagine how many opportunities there are to misspell something just within this page. Further, there are more complex defects—whole sections of the BCRA1 gene may be missing. (Imagine two and a half chapters just deleted from the middle of Tom Sawyer.)

Most genetic screens are designed to find only one specific misspelling or deletion. This leads to the frustrating reality that a donor could undergo 4 or 5 different tests for a BCRA1 mutation—passing each one—and still have the defect.

Donor screening thus becomes a classical case of diminishing returns:
- $1,000 worth of screening eliminates 50 percent of the risk;
- $9,000 more spent on screening eliminates another 40 percent;
- $90,000 is needed to eliminate 5 percent more.

In the end, there is only one way to fully document the genetic risk of a donor. That is to sequence all 6 billion bases in his diploid genome. While this may not be beyond our reach in the near future, for the present, it is prohibitively expensive. Only one person, J. Craig Venter of the Human Genome Project, has been fully sequenced.

What Does This Mean for Donors?

Arguably, naive donors who have been screened for nothing come to the clinic with a defect risk of 2 percent. That is a ballpark number derived from the fact that, generally, about 4 percent of neonates are found to suffer from some genetic condition, and, for simplicity's sake, we will simply split the blame equally among the sexes.

Each act of screening, whether it is limited sequencing, a karyotype, a cystic fibrosis SNP test, or a careful family history, should act to reduce the risks by limiting the door pool to donors who are less likely than the population average to pass along genetic diseases. The amount of risk reduction is directly proportional to the intensity of the screening and the resources expended on it.

Although I support reform of U.S. sperm banks, there is a serious intellectual lapse reflected by the Dutch parliament in response to the ADCA tragedy: the presumption that limiting donors to 10 live births reduces risk.

In fact, the change simply increases the cost of donor semen without changing risk at all.

Since the resources spent qualifying a Dutch donor can only be amortized across 10 children, one must charge the DI parents 1/10 of the screening cost. One must then incur the expense a second time to qualify a new donor who passes the same set of tests when the first donor needs to be retired. This new donor, however, might ultimately suffer from a different undetected genetic illness than the first.

Over time, the Dutch response will potentially result in offspring in smaller clusters, coming from different donors, with different diseases.

As an added concern, two years after the introduction of this law, there are 70 percent fewer semen donors and 50 percent fewer sperm banks in the Netherlands.

The reason so few donors "make the cut" at sperm banks is that, in addition to meeting height, appearance, education and medical background criteria of prospective parents, the donor also needs to have high sperm counts and freeze viability, among other positive fertilization factors necessary for conception. (In fact, it's no wonder that infertility is now recognized to affect 1 out of 10 couples, since there are so many physiological obstacles to overcome.)

To arbitrarily disqualify the relatively rare group of donors that are most successful would further exacerbate the cost of donor semen.

So how might Dutch legislators have done better?

ADCA is a polyglutamine repeat disease with at least 12 variants. In layman's term, the ADCA gene is a book of about 3,000 pages, and while most of the billions of copies of this book on the planet are spelled correctly, perhaps one in 20,000 contain one of 12 possible misspelled words.

Sequencing each donor for ADCA means simply that we would first read the ADCA book (gene) and then submit it to a computer spell-check. One could mandate that all 12 misspelled words (loci) be spell-checked (fully sequenced) for all donors, which would have some interesting consequences. There would be no more donor transmission of ADCA.

Donor semen safety would have been increased ever so slightly by the elimination of this one risk. However, ADCA is a very rare genetic disease, one among hundreds of thousands of known genetic defects. The fact that this disease was passed to offspring by a semen donor catapulted it into media prominence. That by no means implies that it is the most important or cost-effective condition that one could screen in a donor.

And in fact, this new luxury for recipients would come at some substantial increase in cost. The only way to defray this cost would be to spread it out over more inseminations.

This guides us to the conclusion: As genetic testing becomes more stringent, making donor semen safer, the number of inseminations per donor must be allowed to increase in order to offset the increased cost.

The Dutch could have mandated the screening of a handful of the more common transmissible genetic conditions (i.e., cystic fibrosis, Tay-Sachs, Fragile X) and then rewarded the banks by allowing them to use these high-qualified donors for an unlimited number of live births. Instead, many argue that prolific donors should be retired just because they are prolific — that there should be a childbirth limit.

To me, this is based on an ethical concern: How many offspring to any one person makes us feel "queasy?" Whereas science would tell us, starting with Darwin, that only the strongest survive—and in the area of reproductive technology, where science is an inherent part of the process, why wouldn't we want to take advantage of available genetic testing to create the strongest pool that we can? Even if that means having greater numbers of families selecting from the more limited pool of candidates?

When donors should be retired

In the secretive past, it could be argued that donors should be retired to avoid incest among their offspring. That's not a persuasive argument now. DI children should simply be told the names and generic geographic locations of their half siblings, making the point moot.

> *The idea of complete anonymity will die a slow and grudging death, but it runs contrary to the best interests of the children, to public safety, and to sperm bank accountability.*

All donors do not insist on anonymity — in the past, donors like me were simply informed of it. In the future, they simply need to be told that it will not be possible.

There are only few genetic defects that seem to be a consequence of paternal age. The increased risk of schizophrenia in children conceived by men above 50 is the best documented. If a donor's sperm continues to survive with appropriate motility and quantity after freezing, the age of the donor should not be a major issue. And, of course, frozen sperm from previous donation can survive well into the future. A donor's sperm today can be thawed for use in an insemination at least 10 years from now. (Probably even 50 or 100, but no one has felt comfortable testing the limits yet.)

As the donor ages, retirement becomes a rather thorny cost/benefit analysis. If one has spent $60,000 over 25 years, and successfully eliminated 500 genetic illnesses from one donor's pedigree, when is it cost effective to start with a new 25-year-old donor and spend another $60,000?

That's hard to say, since the several hundred healthy offspring that the older donor will likely have over time is the best predictor of his true genetic risk. Even with $60,000 worth of genetic testing, there are still 40,000 or so disease genes that will not have been eliminated.

For me it is clear that comprehensive postnatal follow up of all DI children must be mandated by law—and the information be shared privately with other related families, and anonymously with prospective clients.

If a donor is exceeding a 3 percent birth defect rate — just under the national average — after a statistically significant number of births, he should be retired.

If he is helping families produce strong, healthy, intelligent children, I believe he should be retained and allowed to continue to provide donor semen for many years.

Kirk Maxey was a donor for 15 years. He launched Cayman Chemical, which now employs 240 in drug development and research. His non-profit, Cayman Biomedical Research Institute, focuses on issues of personal interest to him, including the donor insemination industry.

CONCLUSION
By Mikki Morrissette, Editor

The difficulty of compiling a collection of essays such as this is that no one parent, donor or offspring can speak for everyone in their "group." Yet the actual gathering of voices with perspectives to share would be so vast that no one book could do any of them justice. That is why only a handful of thoughtful, articulate voices were picked for this volume: to engage discussion, ask questions and propose (sometimes controversial) suggestions. Not to conclude the debate.

So it is with this Conclusion. It is impossible to sum up the conversations that are debated about these issues—on the Donor Sibling Registry, with my Choice Mom discussion group, between spouses behind closed doors, among industry representatives, even within these pages. Although there are many opinions, there is no neat and tidy list of comprehensive recommendations to offer. There is no "one size fits all" for something as complex as how we build and define our families.

But there are things we can attempt to agree on.

1. We can recognize the deep shame and fear that many infertile parents feel and work toward making it less of a stigma by talking more openly about it, as Eric Schwartzman has done.

2. We can recognize that a parent's fear of being replaced by a donor in the child's eyes—while discounted by offspring—is understandable, based largely on the mixed message from society that biology trumps nurturing as a parental prerequisite for fulfilling a child's needs, and that bloodlines historically mean

something about a person's worth and place.

3. We can acknowledge that a parent's fear does not go away simply by not talking about it, or by hiding it and letting the child believe there is a biological connection that does not exist.

4. We can acknowledge that donor-conceived children grow up to be adults who remember the nurturing of their parents, yet who also have legitimate curiosities about their biological heritage and medical history.

If we agree on those basic points, I think one resolution that should be relatively simple to address is building a communications strategy that starts the moment prospective parents walk into a fertility clinic or place an order for donor sperm, and the moment a prospective donor steps into a bank.

> *An awareness-building campaign, at the "point of purchase" and "point of sale," would bring up the questions that should be examined about the long-term implications and emotional consequences of this choice— for parents, for donors, and for children.*

Each parent and donor would still be free to reach the conclusions that best suit their situation, but a concerted effort would be made to be sure that the questions were asked before conception or donation occurs. For example:

• The names of local mental health specialists in reproductive technology could be provided to consult as a prerequisite, along with literature that explains the reasons why.

• A mandatory workshop, such as that offered by adoption agencies, could be offered to explore the issues publicly.

• A private informational session could be required that covers the impact of this choice on marital relationships, what it entails to tell or not tell family and friends, and how to establish the environment that best serves the needs of the child.

• The often sterile environment of sperm banks could include posters of children in the hallway, to help drive home the point that what happens inside the masturbatorium leads to real human beings.

Simple, effective tools that state out loud important issues.

Why Build Awareness?

So why now? Why a change in policy? Why put the pressure on clinics and sperm banks to require counseling, when all they want to do is help people get pregnant?

The industry has been transformed in recent decades, as Kirk Maxey pointed out in the previous essay. Like adoption, donor insemination is emerging from a less enlightened time when "go home, make love, pretend it's your child" was the wisdom of the day.

There are some who would argue that it was a simpler time when parents kept the truth to themselves and children didn't have the rights we give them today. When it was clear that Mom and Dad and Child were the family unit, not mixed up with half-siblings and donor fathers and surrogates. Why mandate opening up a Pandora's box of questions that can't easily be answered? Why not simply allow parents to work things out on their own, rather than complicate an industry with the messiness of family dynamics?

Three reasons, not even including a basic discussion of ethics.

1. Change in clientele

A growing percentage of people purchasing donor sperm—indeed, half at some banks—are single women or lesbian couples, who have no real need to be secretive or ashamed of donor conception. Sales of donor sperm to married couples has dropped proportionally, partly attributable to new technologies that can sometimes extract working sperm from infertile husbands.

With this new marketplace of open consumers come new challenges. Children who know they are conceived from donor sperm tend to be curious about the donor as a real person, rather than a vial of product. As child development expert Kyle Pruett once told me, "Having useful information about the donor has a way of keeping the child's identity secure. They aren't aliens, created from Kryptonite."

It is the open parents and naturally curious children who are putting pressure on the industry. And to a great extent, sperm banks have complied by providing more extensive donor profiles, multi-generational medical histories, photographs, audiotaped interviews. Sometimes this is sufficient. But very often it is not a substitute for being able to absorb the person, as the three donor-conceived offspring in this book have aptly explained.

Even when children grow up with loving parents, it doesn't negate their longing to "own" their heritage. As Rebecca Hamilton wrote, "If the desire for a biological connection is strong enough to make adults choose donor conception over adoption, then it is the ultimate double standard to imagine that the desire for a biological connection will not be felt just as strongly by the donor-conceived person that results."

As many couples can attest, it's a struggle to keep the secret. And a half-open, half-closed marketplace is difficult to satisfy, as many industry reps can attest. An alternative to proactively advising all parents, in advance of conception, about the deeply felt longing of many children to have an open-identity connection with their donor is to go back to a time when secrecy was advised to all parents, train them how to maintain the secret from everyone without affecting relationships with each other and their child, teach them how to hide the awkward moments when the child picks up clues, and cut off the sizeable market of single mothers and lesbian couples who use donor insemination to build families.

The embryo created with the help of a fertility doctor and/or sperm bank might not grow into a questioning adult, but the ones that do will not easily adhere to a policy of anonymity that others agreed to. Many of them feel strongly that they own the right to their own birth story, their own lineage. And like adoptive children who search for birth family, the coming generations of donor-conceived offspring will have a greater set of tools for finding people they want to find.

Donors today should particularly be made aware that their anonymity is not guaranteed after their offspring grow up.

2. Genetics

The second reason an awareness-building campaign, rather than an openness-diminishing strategy, is inevitable is that scientific innovations make it increasingly beneficial for individuals to know their medical background in order to lead healthier lives. It is increasingly unfair to deny that information to them.

The three-generation histories that many donors provide when they are 20 and unaware is inadequate. Not only is misinformation to be expected, but there is no system to track the truthfulness of the young man who doesn't want to be disqualified from an "easy, well-paying job" because his father takes heart medication.

Also, importantly, even the most accurate medical background forms do not include the donor's "history" that has not been revealed yet—such as the breast cancer the man's mother might battle in 10 years time.

Some geneticists predict that DNA tests will be commonplace in doctor's offices in 10 or 15 years. Thanks to the DNA mapping databases maintained by groups like the National Human Genome Research Institute, an individual's genetic sequencing will be increasingly used to spot patterns and predict trends. With individualized medicine, doctors can design treatments and drugs to work with a person's specific genetic make-up, as well as predict whether a person could develop a particular disease.[1]

For example, blood sent in for one test can reveal if a particular gene has a mutation that makes the person more susceptible to breast and ovarian cancer. Each person inherits a copy of the breast cancer gene (BRCA) from the mother and father, which work in combination to prevent the cancers—unless one of those genes is altered.

The test is costly. It makes sense for people to take it if they are at greater risk, such as those of Ashkenazi/Eastern European Jewish heritage, and those with a family history of breast cancer. There are preventative measures that can be taken to reduce risk if the mutated gene is found, such as more vigilant breast exams, mammograms starting at age 25, ultrasounds to check ovaries, even ovary removal.

Many women who have the mutated gene—which means they have a 60 percent to 85 percent chance of developing breast cancer—elect to have a preventive mastectomy. Men who have the gene are at a higher risk of prostate cancer and male breast cancer.

Many hereditary diseases require the same foresight. CBS News ran the story of one 67-year-old woman whose heart transplant has likely enabled her to survive cardiomyopathy, which killed her mother and three brothers at an earlier age. Because of her known history, her grandchildren already know they carry the gene, and precautions are being taken.

The good news is that as genetic testing becomes more common, less expensive and more accurate in the decades ahead, people who do not know their full genetic background will be able to unlock necessary clues from their own DNA sequencing, without involving the donor.

But prevention is only as good as the medical history available. Someone who has a history of depression from the donor's side, for example, deserves to know. Today there are genetic tests available for roughly 1,000 diseases, which allow doctors to diagnose disease, predict risk, and guide decisions about treatments. No individual can take every test, which is why it is still beneficial to know of hereditary factors as a warning.

The growing field of DNA testing also means that unexplained paternity will more easily be revealed. This is not limited to medicine. Molecular genealogy is a burgeoning area of interest for amateur and professional family historians, who can learn interesting details from a simple swab of the cheek.

One man I heard about, active in genealogical research, submitted his DNA results into a database search engine and learned that he was closely linked to a family surname that was not his father's. He learned that his biological father was not the father listed on his birth certificate. Further research revealed that he descended from a particular family in his mother's hometown.

3. Bad public relations

No amount of genetic screening can detect every anomaly in a donor's bloodline. For one, often it takes mutations, or a combination of genes from mother and father, or more than a single base pair to be adversely affected. Also, any number of genetic diseases are not tested, and it would be prohibitively expensive to run the hundreds available.

Sperm banks are getting into trouble, however, largely because of a breakdown in communication with purchasers of their product after the genetics of the donor are called into question. National media attention has pointed out cases such as these:

> • In "The Truth About Donor 1048" (*Self* magazine, October 2006), several case studies were compiled of angry mothers who believed sperm banks were hiding evidence of donors' genetic defects. One case involved four families who used the same donor; their children at a young age reportedly all suffer from eczema, allergies and asthma. According to the article, what particularly bothered the mothers was that the sperm bank did not report potential issues involving that donor to other families or prospective parents.

> • In August 2006, Associated Press reported a story nationwide about four families with a shared donor whose children all had signs of autism. The MSNBC headline read, "Banks don't disclose

medical information, so moms seek answers elsewhere." Although the article pointed out that it is not yet known whether autism is a hereditary disease, the primary accusation was that the mothers had been unable to find out more about the donor's history.

• In May 2006, *The Journal of Pediatrics* reported a case involving at least five children of one donor who inherited congenital neutropenia. Analysis of the donor's sperm could not be done without his permission, and the sperm bank had been unable to find him, or warn him that he risked passing the disease on to his own children.

If the industry encouraged a more open relationship between providers of product (donors) and purchasers of product (parents), sperm banks in particular might not get into such trouble as the liaison responsible for keeping families and donors anonymous.

Families who prefer to have access to medical updates from others who use the same donor, and from the donor directly, could be asked to participate in a database that would not only track births from the same man, but allow all of those parties to have anonymous contact with each other related to medical issues that come up over time.

There have been several people—ranging from bioethicists, mental health counselors, newspaper editorial writers, parents, lawyers, and others involved in behind-the-scenes conversations—talking about how to make this kind of database happen.

For all of these reasons, it makes sense that an awareness-building campaign needs to be developed that brings all parties to the table in an effort to create effective tools that usher the industry into the new world it is destined to be.

What would a campaign involve?

An awareness-building campaign is not difficult to implement. But it does require a willingness to develop a new strategy around donation and purchase:

• Donors need to be made aware of the kinds of questions offspring will have of them, and why, and be willing to make their sperm and limited contact information available to a certain number of families, perhaps staggered over time.

• Families who want their children to have the option of knowing the donor need to be willing to make themselves known to him in advance as well, so that he can be as aware of them over time as they will be of him.

• Legal protections need to be put in place so that donors and families can negotiate contact—when, how, expectations—similar to the discussions many Choice Moms have with known donors.

Not all donors and parents will be willing to go this route. Choices will be available, as they are today. But an awareness-building campaign, over time, at the point of purchase or donation, would not allow people to walk into reproduction with third-party gametes without a much greater comprehension of what that entails, for themselves and the children.

Some recipients have used the enhanced profile information about anonymous donors to track them down later. If more recipients understood the strong curiosity and urge to "know more"—for themselves or their children—at the front end, instead of focusing all attention on conceiving, they could be steered toward using an open-identity donor instead of impinging on the privacy of donors who may or may not welcome contact. (After all, as one sperm bank director told me, we wouldn't want donors tracking offspring at will.)

By opening up discussion at the front end of the "business transaction," the goal is to save a lot of the emotional aftershocks that inevitably occur.

The Downsides of Awareness

Many families, of course, don't want to welcome strangers—even biologically connected ones—into their life. Undoubtedly some who become more aware before conception occurs will shy away from donor insemination as an option. But personally, I do not think that is a "bad" thing.

Others will recognize that deeper conversation is required to reduce the fears they face by making this choice.

As Wendy Kramer points out, parents might have clear limits on who is important and who is not, but their donor-conceived children might not have the same parameters over time. Some prospective parents might need to share out loud their definition of family, and what would happen if others—such as their child or spouse—eventually had a different definition.

Discomfort is to be expected, of course. Eric Schwartzman did not listen to the audiotaped interviews with his donor for several years. And as he readily admits, he feels threatened by and jealous of the existence of a man he does not know who has a permanent connection to his children.

But there is a big difference between being aware of the donor as a person and being able to talk about him—as Eric does—and shutting out acknowledgement and conversation about the donor's existence.

Listen in on conversations on the Donor Sibling Registry on any given day for a reminder of how emotional it is to be aware of this distinction.

Many donors, of course, don't want to welcome strangers—even biologically connected ones—into their life either. Undoubtedly some who become more aware will shy away from sperm donation as an option. But personally, I do not think that is a "bad" thing either.

As three professionals who offer fertility services in Manchester, U.K., wrote in a commentary that appeared in the online publication BioNews, they have been successful in donor recruitment—even after the laws changed in 2006 to offer only open-identity donors—by changing attitudes about the process.[2]

As they wrote, they recognized a new strategy in donor recruitment was required to find men willing to be identified in the future. A news and current affairs magazine in the U.K. written by professionals, with proceeds going to help the homeless, had led to half of their donors. Inquiries on donation are handled quickly and personally, rather than simply sending out information packets. When donor testing begins, detailed information is discussed about the process, the responsibilities, the importance of details about family history.

"The profiles of identifiable donors are different to previous donors," they wrote. "As anticipated they are older, mostly in employment and quite often have families of their own, compared with the younger, generally student, anonymous donors. Gone are the days where sperm donation was regarded as 'beer money.' Nowadays we need to encourage men to come forward and commit themselves to a lengthy but rewarding process. We must treat them with the respect they deserve. We certainly do not have a shortage of potential donors in Manchester, but donor recruitment requires a dedicated team who recognise and support the wisdom underlying the change in the law."

Other Voices

This Voices of Donor Conception series was launched because there seems to be a huge gap of understanding between many involved in the industry (doctors, sperm bank representatives) and the people affected by the industry (donors, parents, offspring). This first volume is an attempt to bridge that gap. It is in no way comprehensive of the many questions to be answered, or of the many voices and personal stories available, or of the views on the issues.

This volume was focused, as narrowly as possible, on opening up discussion by bringing fears, frustrations, and regrets out from behind closed doors and into the daylight. The momentum of public dialogue about these issues needs to continue to build—involving doctors, mental health counselors, lawyers, bioethicists, sperm bank directors, parents, donors, offspring, legislators.

A pending title in this book series is *Making Contact*, which gets into the honest ups and downs of donors, parents and offspring who make contact with each other:

• The wife of a donor who is being contacted by grown offspring, and how that makes her feel as the mother of their two young children;

• An anonymous donor who did not want contact, and why, but was located from information in his extended profile, as well as the reasons why the parent made contact;

• A couple that does not agree about whether to make contact with half-siblings of their donor-conceived children, and advice about how to handle that division;

• Half-siblings who have met and found great joy in adding to their family network, others who didn't find the experience as profound;

• Do's and don'ts for reaching out.

Another possible title in the series, *The Business of Sperm*, would look at the industry from the perspective of sperm bank directors, such as:

• Why directors of smaller banks are getting squeezed out of business, and what impact they think it will have on the market;

• When a bank claims that its donors reduce the risk of cervical cancer to recipients, or that its open-identity donors will be reachable someday, or that a limited number of offspring are allowed, who validates those claims?

• How The Sperm Bank of California keeps communication open between its donors, parents and offspring over time.

Other questions that could be explored:

• Do children with no siblings seem to have more interest in making contact with donors and half-siblings?

• How do people maintain privacy about their method to parenthood, without overburdening children and others with the need for secrecy?

• Should recipients be screened as part of the matching process with particular donors?

• Is government intervention necessary in regulating the industry, or to be avoided?

• Should donor insemination become less expensive, since infertility does not discriminate based on income level? Or should it become more expensive, to enable greater availability of open, highly screened donors? Is today's system a happy medium?

The goal of Voices of Donor Conception will be to encourage open, rational discussion between parties on all sides of the table, in order to commit to finding solutions that work, one step at a time. It is not to try to convince everyone of a "right" side—other than the prevailing intent to bring donor-conceived children into the forefront of considerations, rather than simply focusing on the conception process.

ENDNOTES

[1] There are many good sources of information about the future of genetic testing. One interesting article is "Fast Forward to 2020: What to Expect in Molecular Medicine," by Daniel Drell (U.S. Department of Energy) and Anne Adamson (Oak Ridge National Laboratory), which speculates about how genetic advances related to the Human Genome Project might affect the practice of medicine in the next 20 years. It originally appeared in the online magazine TNTY Futures.

[2] The commentary about progressive donor recruitment practices was written by Joanne Adams, Senior Andrologist, Manchester Fertility Services; Dr. Elizabeth Pease, Consultant in Reproductive Medicine, St Mary's Hospital, Manchester; Professor Brian Lieberman, Medical Director, Manchester Fertility Services. It appeared in BioNews 16 October 2006 (www.bionews.org.uk)

INCLUDE YOUR VOICE

The Voices of Donor Conception book series will continue to share honest stories and strong viewpoints to help inform the conversation.

Suggestions for themes, and stories, are welcomed at
DCVoices@gmail.com.

To offer a viewpoint that extends from this Voices of Donor Conception conversation, contact **DCVoices@yahoogroups.com.**

You'll also find many of these themes discussed in an ongoing way at
www.DonorSiblingRegistry.com

Visit **www.VoicesofDonorConception.com** for updates, additional insight, and more related to this book series.

THIS COLLECTION OF STORIES WAS COMPILED
AS A COLLABORATION BETWEEN:

Wendy Kramer
wwwDonorSiblingRegistry.com

As one-half of an infertile couple, Wendy Kramer's son Ryan was conceived in 1989 with the help of anonymous donor insemination. She has raised him as a single parent since he was one. Unable to satisfy his curiosity by making contact with half-siblings through the sperm bank, they turned to the Internet when Ryan was 10. Since posting the first Donor Sibling Registry message in September 2000, the site has become a hub for donor families. Wendy has communicated extensively with donor-conceived offspring, parents, donors, family members, researchers, educators, and health professionals. She is currently partnering with a Cambridge University research team on a groundbreaking study about the effects of searching and finding donor relatives. Wendy and Ryan have talked about the donor insemination business on Good Morning America, The Today Show, The Early Show, CNN, PBS, BBC, NPR, The Oprah Winfrey Show, 60 Minutes, and on behalf of The New York Times, Washington Post, London Times, and many others.

Mikki Morrissette
www.ChoosingSingleMotherhood.com

Mikki Morrissette is the mother of two children conceived with a known donor. She is author of *Choosing Single Motherhood: The Thinking Woman's Guide,* which has sold in ten countries, and moderates an international discussion group for Choice Moms. She is not only a respected and authoritative voice to the Choice Mom community, which makes up half of the donor insemination industry's clientele, but she has an extensive background as writer and editor in tackling challenging material in a comprehensive and non-threatening way. As a long-time communications consultant, for places ranging from Time Inc. to The New York Times, with clients ranging from Girl Scouts to financial institutions, she launched Be-Mondo Publishing to bridge gaps of understanding between individuals and institutions.